YOUR BLOOD AND ITS PRESSURE

J. I. Rodale

and The Editors of *Prevention*

RODALE BOOKS, INC.

Emmaus, Penna. 18049

Standard Book Number 87596-043-X
Library of Congress Catalog Card Number 73-104180

Printed in United States
SECOND PRINTING — NOVEMBER, 1971
PB-54

Table of Contents

Part Three:
Guidelines for a Healthy Circulatory System

Introduction

WITH FRIGHTENING FREQUENCY we read these days of young men in their 20's and 30's who, without warning, are overcome with fatal heart attacks. A 24-year-old high school football coach, believed in excellent physical condition, leaves the field after a workout, goes to his car, and minutes later is found dead, slumped over the wheel. A 32-year-old athlete suddenly keels over while jogging through a city park, a victim of a fatal coronary infarction. Their hearts have failed, but it is the diseased condition of their blood vessels that has caused the failure.

It is certainly true that people have always died of heart attacks—and anyone who wishes to press the issue might insist that everyone who dies does so because his heart stops beating. But the point is that today atherosclerotic heart disease—a disease hardly known 50 years ago—kills more of us than any other disease. For the truth of the matter is that, if the trend continues as it has in recent years, statistical averages tell us that either you or your spouse will die from cardiovascular disease, probably caused by blockage of the arteries.

Incredible as that fact may be, even more incredible is this one: the major heart diseases—those that take their yearly toll of millions—can be prevented! Evidence for this statement has been gathering for several years now—in fact, from the time that heart disease was recognized by the medical community as a major cause of death. Medical libraries across the country are stacked with tons of literature on how you can prevent or reduce clogging of the arteries, control blood pressure, improve circulation and in other ways prevent the major causes of injury to the heart and brain.

As one doctor put it, "Based on the information we now have, no one need ever die of a heart attack!" The same is not equally true of the sudden cerebrovascular hemorrhages that cause most strokes, yet many of these could also be prevented.

But that information has remained all too long on those stuffy medical library shelves. And men and women continue to die, day after day and year after year, in appalling numbers.

This book has been written to bring the information out of the library and into your hands. Here you will find a clear discussion of your body's circulatory system—how it functions, what can interfere with its smooth operation, and what diseases can occur. You will read the latest in both fact and theory about how these diseases can be avoided and have been in many cases. This book is intended to be a practical guide to circulatory system health for you and your family.

But a healthy circulatory system does not come about through reading. In fact, sitting in an easy chair with a book in your lap for too many hours a day can be detrimental. This book will tell you how you may improve your health in this respect. That's all. And merely knowing how to do something never helped anybody.

The final steps must be taken by you. Unless you truly determine to implement the information between these covers, it can be no more valuable to you than if it had remained on the library shelves. And so this book has a dual purpose—not only to present you with facts you will need to maintain and improve your health, but to prod you and to inspire you to put those facts to work in your life every day and every minute.

—The Editors

BLOOD PRESSURE AND THE CIRCULATORY SYSTEM

Part One: The Blood Vessels

CHAPTER I

Description of the Circulatory System

ALTHOUGH the earliest physicians recognized the fact that the human body contains miles of tubes whose function is to pump nourishing blood throughout the nervous system, it is only in relatively recent times that we have begun to understand the diseases of the body's plumbing system and how to prevent them.

An Englishman named William Harvey was the first person who clearly described the circulation and, in 1628, proved it by experimentation. Following Harvey, Professor Bellini of Pisa, Italy, noted that arteries become hardened and blocked, thus anticipating recognition of the heart's chief diseases.

In 1782, William Heberden wrote the classic description of angina pectoris, commenting that attacks could be brought on by "any disturbance of mind." About this time, a Shropshire "wise woman" called Old Mother Hutton became known for healing brew that she prepared for her practice of folk medicine in the countryside. William Withering studied the potions Old Mother Hutton used and found they contained foxglove, a common plant. He further discovered that this plant had a stimulating effect on the heart. Today we know that the active ingredient of foxglove is digitalis, which is widely used—and misused—in the treatment of disorders of the circulatory system.

Components of the Blood

Life began in the sea, and the red fluid that bathes the cells of our body is very much like sea water. It forms an "inside environment" for us that normally remains constant whether it rains or snows, whether we sweat or shiver.

Our blood contains red cells that carry oxygen and carbon dioxide, white blood cells that swim into action to fight off infection, and blood platelets that help maintain the fluidity of circulating blood and provide the ingredients needed for the blood clot in case of injury.

In addition to these formed elements of the blood, there are soluble elements, such as enzymes, protective antibodies, hormones, organic products such as urea, ammonia, sugar and amino acids—the "building blocks" of protein. We also find inorganic salts of sodium, calcium, potassium, phosphorus and iron, as well as various trace elements and various serum proteins that help regulate blood volume and assist in clotting.

An adult possesses about a quart of blood (one thousand cc.) for each 25 pounds of body weight. Slightly more than half the total quantity of circulating blood is a clear fluid called plasma. And although plasma is about 92 percent water, it carries substances vital to our existence, such as red blood cells or erythrocytes (ee-rith-row-sites), white blood cells or leucocytes (luke-oh-sites), and platelets or thrombocytes (throm-bow-sites).

Most of us are familiar with red and white blood corpuscles, but clotting requires a third kind of corpuscle. These are called platelets because they are shaped like tiny plates.

The red blood cells are the most numerous, amounting to about 30 trillion in the average person. Each cell lives three or four months and is then eliminated or reconstituted. This means that millions upon millions of red blood cells are being scrapped and reconstituted every minute of every hour, day and night.

The red cells hold an iron-containing substance called hemoglobin that picks up oxygen when it passes through the lungs and carries this life-giving gas to tissues throughout the body.

The white blood cells are two to three times larger than the red, but there are not so many of them. For the most part, they are manufactured in the bone marrow and increase greatly when an infection attacks.

Another part of the internal environment is a fluid, much like blood plasma, called lymph. It oozes through the walls of the smallest blood vessels, bathes the cells and tissue constantly, and carries away waste products. You have often seen lymph in a water blister on your skin.

Your blood keeps the cells of your body bathed at all times with a constant amount of fluid containing balanced amounts of chemicals at even temperatures. Of course all the organs of the body affect and are affected by the blood. Lungs, intestines, kidneys, liver, glands, and many more organs all must do their part.

When the blood carries sugar thoughout the body at a steady rate of one part glucose to a thousand parts of blood, it does so by virtue of being able to unload excess sugar on the liver. The liver, in turn, releases sugar as the cells use it up, or changes it to fat and stores it under the skin, in the marrow of the bones, around the kidneys, and elsewhere.

If the blood should be overloaded with sugar for some reason, the kidneys go to work to wash it out fast.

Blood also carries a supply of salt, and this changes even less than the sugar content. The kidneys also unload excess salt, but they lose water in doing so. The water comes from the blood which borrowed it from the cells. So now you begin to feel thirsty until you drink some more water, which is returned to the blood and cells.

The blood also regulates its own acidity. The cells of the body are constantly pouring acids into the blood, which neutralizes them and maintains a strict balance.

The vessels that carry the blood are often likened to pipes that carry water in a city. The analogy holds insofar as the blood vessels form a branching system that starts at a central main (the heart) and divides and sub-divides into smaller and smaller pipes.

But the blood vessels are not metal pipes or glass tubes. They are truly flesh and blood, and they remain soft and elastic as the fluid flows through them.

There are three different kinds of blood vessels: arteries, veins and capillaries. Each of them is adapted to do a special job. Arteries carry fresh blood, reinforced with oxygen from the lungs, to the various parts of the body. The veins pick up the used blood and return it for reoxygenation. The capillaries link the two systems.

The large arteries are like thick rubber hoses and are made up of three layers, like tubes enclosed by other tubes. Under a microscope you can see that the thin lining layer called the *intima* is made of flat, very smooth cells. Another thin layer of loose fibers surrounds this inner lining and is called the *media.* Finally, the outside coating, called the *adventitia,* is made up of connective tissue.

All the larger arteries have similar structure. Smaller arteries, called arterioles, also have three layers but are not replicas of the larger arteries. The main difference is in the middle layer. This is elastic tissue in the larger arteries, but mostly muscle in the smaller ones.

This difference is important to an understanding of disorders of the circulatory system. The large arteries are strong enough easily to withstand the pressure of the blood pumped by the heart. Moreover, they stretch to accommodate the blood for an instant and then squeeze back to their narrower width. This amounts to giving the heart an assist in pushing the blood along to the smaller arteries.

The arterioles work a bit differently. While they also widen and tighten, they do not do so in rhythm with the heart but, rather, as called upon by the body. For example, if you begin to exercise strenuously, the small arteries will open wide so that additional blood flows to the hard-working muscles.

The capillaries, unlike the arteries, have walls so thin that they are made of only one layer of cells. They are not very strong, but they do not need to be because by the time the blood reaches them it has lost about two-thirds of its pressure. This is why you needn't worry about the capillaries bursting under normal circumstances. Actually, they are so thin that the fluid part of the blood can ooze through them into the spaces around the cells.

The capillaries can be considered as irrigation tubes carrying water and dissolved food to the tissue. Like tiny filters, they let out the watery part of the blood in which the food substances have been broken down into their chemical substances, while they keep larger particles such as unbrokendown proteins.

Most important, the capillaries link the tiniest branches of the arteries with the tiny veins.

The veins have thicker walls than the capillaries but thinner than the arteries. The walls of the veins also show three layers but with less muscle and more strands of white fibers. By the time the blood reaches the veins, of course, its pressure is even less than in the capillaries. A tiny vein can drain a whole network of capillaries and then merge into larger and larger veins. This is the opposite of what happens in the arteries: when leaving the heart, the blood is pumped through arteries that become increasingly smaller.

One more important difference between veins and arteries: veins have valves, arteries do not. The valves are necessary because the pressure in the veins is so low that the blood wouldn't have enough push to get back to the heart if the little valves didn't catch it and hold it and help it upstream as it climbs from the feet back up to the abdomen and heart.

This description of the blood and blood vessels is obviously quite oversimplified. To discuss it in detail would take a book all by itself. What it contains is the basic information needed to a clearer understanding of how to prevent disorders in these marvelous mechanisms of the human body.

CHAPTER II

Blood Pressure

THE FORCE of the blood against the walls of the blood vessels as it flows through the body is called the blood pressure. The pressure is created by the pumping of the heart. In "reading" the blood pressure, we use two sets of numbers—one for when the heart contracts (the systolic pressure) and one for when it is at rest (diastolic pressure).

For example when we say the blood pressure is 140 over 80, we mean that when the heart is in systole, the pressure will push a column of mercury to the 140 mark on the blood pressure measuring instrument. When the heart rests between beats, the pressure drops to a diastolic reading of 80.

The systolic pressure varies greatly and is affected by nervousness, excitement and exertion. In fact, the mere act of having the blood pressure taken in a doctor's office upsets some people so that their pressure rises. But in a little while it is likely to drop again without causing any damage.

The diastolic pressure, on the other hand, remains fairly constant and therefore is the more important reading of the two. People who say "my blood pressure is 180" are usually talking about the systolic pressure.

The old saying that the blood pressure should be "100 plus your age" is not true. What is "normal" for a person varies with age, height, weight, temperament, diet, and many other variables. There is little agreement among doctors concerning "normal" blood pressure, though most of them agree that the diastolic pressure should be viewed with suspicion if it exceeds 90 or falls below 60.

The figures for the systolic pressure would be suspect if the pressure were lower than 110 or higher than 160 or 170. Perhaps the relationship between systolic and diastolic pressures is the important thing. A healthy ratio would be three to two: 150/100, 120/80, etc.

The many variables that affect the blood pressure must always be kept in mind. For example, one's blood pressure may be higher if taken by a strange doctor—and if the doctor himself is tense or irritable he may affect the reading.

Your blood pressure is higher when sitting or lying down, lower when erect. It is inclined to be higher in stocky people, lower in lanky ones—and is greatly affected by overweight.

So it is possible for a person with a basically normal systolic pressure to be diagnosed as a "hypertensive" in a hospital or doctor's office, or under unusual circumstances, whereas under more favorable conditions his pressure would be considered well within normal. And, of course, once certain people have the name, they also "have the game;" that is, the falsely diagnosed "hypertensive" becomes a victim of anxiety about his heart (cardiophobia) and his pressure shoots higher. Thus, an original inadequate diagnosis is compounded and carried on.

Under such conditions, a statistician who says "there are ten million high blood pressure victims in the United States" might well be pressed to reveal under just what circumstances the blood pressure readings were taken—and if they adequately reflect the relation between the systolic and diastolic readings.

When a doctor takes your blood pressure, he fastens a cuff containing a rubber bag around your upper arm. By pumping a little rubber bulb he inflates the rubber bag until it squeezes your arm. The doctor listens to your pulse with a stethescope and notes the point at which the bag squeezes hard enough to cut the pulse off.

Then he lets the air out of the bag until he can hear the pulse again. He notes the reading and marks this point as your systolic pressure. He continues to let air out of the bag until the pulse becomes normal again, hardly audible; and this is the diastolic reading.

As we have said, this latter is the more important reading to keep in mind when talking of high and low blood pressures. The medical name for high blood pressure is hypertension. That for low blood pressure hypotension.

High blood pressure is second only to hardening of the arteries as a cause of heart and circulatory diseases in the United States. It is often the real villain behind heart failures, strokes, heart and kidney disease. Yet high blood pressure need not be deadly; it can be prevented or controlled by proper diet, exercise and other means.

One of the prime factors in high blood pressure is one's state of mind. Many people have an unreasoning fear of this condition—and the fear is sometimes worse than the high blood pressure itself. This is why you should understand how the heart and circulatory system work. If you are a heart patient, understanding will help abolish fear and enable you to steer a middle course—neither resigning yourself to the life of an invalid nor stubbornly ignoring a menace to your comfort and longevity.

CHAPTER III

Symptoms of Abnormal Blood Pressure

THE OUTWARD SYMPTOMS of high blood pressure are not always so noticeable that a victim will detect them. Yet there are a number of signals that warn of possible danger, and these should always be investigated. A doctor will not accept symptoms alone as proof of high blood pressure but will conduct a thorough examination.

Frequent headaches are perhaps the most common symptom of high blood pressure. Yet, as we know, headaches can have many causes, some totally unrelated to circulation. They can even be caused by pressure that is too low if, for example, the blood vessels in the brain and other parts of the body have widened, or relaxed unduly, for some reason.

In any case, you should determine if the headaches are due to fluctuations in the blood pressure. If so, study of your diet and manner of living may suggest a cause for the condition, and a preventive diet may alleviate it.

Dizziness or lightheadedness is another common symptom of disorders in the blood pressure and circulatory system. The person affected feels he is going to faint, though he seldom does. There is a difference between dizziness and another symptom of high blood pressure—vertigo. In vertigo there is a sensation that everything in sight is revolving around you or that you are moving somehow. Vertigo is serious, and occasionally "blackouts" occur.

Some people with high blood pressure blush very easily. This can be embarrassing and annoying—but seldom dangerous!

Emotional and physical fatigue are frequently symptoms of high blood pressure. This isn't because there is any definite relationship between tiredness and the height of the blood pressure. It's simply that with the onset of hypertension, which is a disease, people have the usual reaction to sickness and begin to tire more easily. If you fight early fatigue and drive yourself to work as hard as ever, it may be very harmful. If you accept the fatigue as a warning and ease up, you may very well benefit from such a symptom.

Sensations of numbness or tingling in the arms and fingers are not very important in themselves, nor is a feeling of fullness in the head or tightness over the scalp—though these symptoms should be noted and reported to your doctor.

None of these symptoms will tell the degree and nature of the hypertension, or even if it truly exists. A series of blood pressure readings plus examinations of the blood vessels, kidneys, the heart's performance, and other factors are required to make an adequate diagnosis.

Kidney tests are necessary in order to determine what effect the hypertension is having on the body's filtering system. The flow of blood through the kidney is important, as is the amount of functioning tissue.

The progress of high blood pressure is written, literally, on the small blood vessels at the back of the eye. These small vessels are the only blood vessels in the body that can be seen easily and clearly without surgical procedures.

By shining a bright light through a dilated eye pupil, an experienced eye doctor can tell from the condition of these tiny arterioles what damage is being done by hypertension. Periodic eye examinations, therefore, will be more reliable than blood pressure readings to decide how the body is coping with high blood pressure.

The two types of hypertension that occur most frequently are organic hypertension and "essential" or benign hypertension. Neither is the inevitable "killer" that some medical men and drug manufacturers would have us believe.

Organic hypertension is most often acquired and is usually due to detectable disease of the heart, arteries, kidneys or internal secretory glands. It usually gets worse, sometimes slowly, occasionally at such a fast pace that it is called "malignant"—though it has nothing to do with cancer. As organic hypertension progresses, various "target organs" become involved, such as cerebral blood vessels (stroke), coronary arteries (myocardial infarction), kidneys (uremia), or the eyes.

By contrast, no significant disease is detectable in essential hypertension, and it does not progress. It seldom produces secondary symptoms (except anxiety states resulting from misunderstanding and worry about it) and strikes no "target organ."

Low Blood Pressure

Ordinarily, when you stand up, your blood pressure drops from 10 to 20 points. Normally, the heart can handle this without any trouble, and you don't even notice it—although occasionally you could experience just a moment's giddiness.

However, if the blood pressure should drop 30 to 50 points, you might lose consciousness, and your low blood pressure would be called, medically, orthostatic hypotension. This type of low blood pressure is most apt to occur in tall, lanky people —in convalescents after long illness, in fat people who have lost too much weight too rapidly (often due to some punishing diet), in mothers after childbirth, and in those who let their stomach muscles become flabby from lack of exercise.

Low blood pressure is less common and less serious than high blood pressure. But if your diastolic pressure is consistently less than 60, you should have a competent doctor trace the cause and advise you.

Many of the same preventive measures that apply to correcting high blood pressure also work with low blood pressure. Nature always welcomes assistance in preventing illness or restoring health and there is a great deal you can do to provide such assistance.

CHAPTER IV

Disorders of the Circulatory System

ONE OF THE most serious threats to the body is that the arteries supplying it with blood, or the veins draining it, will become clogged or narrowed. Arteriosclerosis and atherosclerosis, which will be discussed in the next chapter, concern the narrowing of the lumen and hardening of the arteries. This condition is probably the major cause of high blood pressure—more force is needed to push the volume of blood through the narrowed and less elastic vessels.

Several kinds of obstructions can occur in the blood vessels, and understanding them can eliminate fear and encourage prevention. Circulatory disturbances affect the heart, brain, kidneys, arms, legs and sometimes the face or parts of it, such as the ears, nose or chin. If enough blood does not reach any of these areas for them to function normally, serious damage may occur.

An interruption in the flow of the blood to the brain for only a half minute will cause unconsciousness. If the interruption is longer, say a minute or two, permanent damage can result. A "stroke" occurs when the blood supply to the brain is cut off by a clot forming in a tiny artery, or by hemorrhage. Hemorrhage occurs where the vessel is too weak to sustain the pressure of the blood.

Clots can also cut off blood to the kidneys, though there the damage is more gradual. If arteries in the arms or legs clog up, the symptoms may be anything from mild pain to swelling, open sores, and loss of the limb due to gangrene. Here we will say a few words about some of the less serious disorders that can nevertheless occasionally bring real trouble. Most of these ailments can be readily prevented.

Buerger's disease, known medically as thromboangiitis obliterans, has been almost exclusively an ailment of the male sex. In recent years, more women have been getting it, probably due to smoking. The condition is an inflammatory process in the blood vessels that produces clots and spreads to the entire circulatory system of the affected parts. Usually, though not always, these are the extremities: hands, toes and feet. If the disease is not stopped, it can end in gangrene. The clots do not form because of accumulations of fat, as in atherosclerosis, but because of inflammation. And they invade the veins as well as the arteries.

The factors causing Buerger's disease are not all known, but it rarely occurs in non-smokers. Frequently the symptoms disappear when patients stop smoking—but come back again if smoking is resumed.

The first symptoms of this disease are very mild, something like a "pins and needles" sensation where the circulation is impaired, or a feeling either of coldness or burning. As the disease progresses, pain sets in and sends the patient to the doctor. The medical advice invariably is common sense: no more smoking.

Raynaud's syndrome (a syndrome is a group of symptoms) is caused by spasm of the smallest arteries, temporarily cutting off the blood supply. The three things that bring this on are cold, emotional disturbance, and the habitual use of vibrating machines such as pneumatic hammers, riveting machines, or polishers.

Why some people are affected while others are not is a mystery. About 70 percent of those who have Raynaud's syndrome are women. It takes a long time before any permanent damage occurs, though it does occur in a few patients. Sores and gangrene may follow, but they usually are confined to the skin. Because of the threat of gangrene, amputations once were common in Raynaud's syndrome. Today such amputations are rare, and in many patients the disease never goes beyond blanching and flushing.

Blocked circulation due to cold can result in frostbite, chilblains, trench foot and immersion foot. Frostbite is a combination of constriction of the arteries and freezing of the fluid that is found between all cells. This freezing causes crystals to form and rupture the cells. Clots tend to form in the smaller arteries, contributing to the breakdown of the tissue.

Frostbite is sometimes related to arterial disease, when partly constricted or blocked blood vessels leave hands and feet susceptible to cold. Trench foot or immersion foot results when soldiers are forced to crouch in trenches or foxholes for days in cold mud, or if survivors of a shipwreck are exposed to cold and soaking for many days.

Diseases of the Veins

Since the walls of veins do not contain as much muscle and elastic tissue as the walls of arteries, they stretch out of shape more easily. Therefore, when clots or inflammation occurs in the veins, bulges develop, producing varicose (dilated) veins. Varicose veins are those whose valves do not hold up adequately. The result is that the blood distends the walls of the veins. Although this usually happens in veins close to the surface in the legs, varicose veins can form anywhere in the body. The legs are the areas most commonly affected by varicose veins, probably because the venous pressure increases with the distance below the heart.

Varicose veins may lead to chronic swelling of the legs during the day, usually at the ankle and lower leg; while lying horizontally during the night, the leg may return to normal. If the condition persists, the skin of the lower legs may darken and develop a type of eczema that causes itching. Again, the skin and tissue just under it may harden and ulcers develop.

A combination of a blood clot and inflammation in a vein is called thrombophlebitis. It is a frequent disorder of the veins and perhaps the most serious which occurs. It is due to a combination of factors.

The inner wall of the vein may become inflamed due to an injury or infection—or even surgery—and may thereby provide favorable conditions for the formation of a clot. Prolonged inactivity for any reason may have a similar effect, which explains why patients are encouraged to get out of bed as soon as possible after surgery and childbirth.

The danger from a clot in a vein is not so much that it will obstruct the flow of blood as that portions of it may break off and be carried in the bloodstream to the lungs, where they may cause serious damage, even death.

Most of these common disorders of the arteries and veins can be prevented or alleviated by adequate preventive measures, as can the major cardiac threats to life, according to competent clinical and research physicians in the field.

CHAPTER V

Hardening of the Arteries

THE MAIN heart artery is the aorta which is about one-half inch to one inch wide at the place where it leaves the left section of the heart and begins to branch out into smaller arteries, which carry blood to the head, the abdomen, the arms, legs and so forth. Women's arteries are wider than men's, possibly because of the greater strains women are called on to endure in childbirth.

The medical term for hardening of the arteries is "arteriosclerosis." The term for narrowing of the arteries due to accumulations of deposits on the inner walls is "atherosclerosis." These terms are sometimes used interchangeably since they are so closely related. Atherosclerosis is one special form of arteriosclerosis.

Hardening of the arteries or arteriosclerosis is a disorder generally associated with growing old, though it occurs quite frequently in people below middle age. It is difficult to diagnose or study, for naturally the process is going on inside the walls of the arteries where it cannot be observed first hand in a living person. However, it is generally accepted that what happens first is a fatty deposit on the inside of the walls which gradually becomes thicker and attracts mineral deposits as well. Now as anyone can see, a hollow tube whose inside walls are heavily crusted with fat and minerals will not continue to supply enough room for the blood to move along at the normal rate. As the space inside the arteries grows smaller, more pressure is exerted on the blood and we have "high blood pressure."

Symptoms may be tingling or cramps, aches or sharp pains when you are using your arms or legs. As the deposits gather on the arteries leading to the brain there may be partial loss of mental ability, disorders of memory and so forth. Of course the arteries leading to the heart itself, the kidneys, the liver and brain are extremely important for good health and the final stages of hardening of the arteries may be complicated with diseases of these organs, since they are simply not receiving enough blood to stay healthy.

As lumps of fatty material collect on artery walls they may project so far into the bloodstream as to form a barrier to the blood flow. Or they may break off in chunks and float around in the blood. When they reach a smaller blood vessel, they become jammed between the walls and a serious condition develops.

What causes hardening of the arteries? Medical authors admit they do not know. Some say it is too much cholesterol in the diet. Cholesterol is a fatty substance that occurs in animal fats, such as milk, butter, fat meat and so forth. Others say that the amount of cholesterol in the diet is not important. The important thing is how the body uses the cholesterol. Why does it deposit on the artery walls in some people and not in others? Is it not something about the whole metabolism of the person, *or something else in the food he may eat,* that protects him from hardening of the arteries?

The Width of Arteries

A most important aspect of the arteries is their width or diameter. This is seldom discussed, even in medical journals, yet it's quite obvious that wide, roomy arteries can carry more blood than narrow ones. This makes the heart's work easier, too.

Osler, the famous physician, once remarked that if one wishes to live long, much depends upon the quality of the arterial tissue, "the vital rubber," as he termed it. The disadvantage of narrow arteries is that if a narrow-arteried person gets cholesterol deposits on the walls of his blood vessels, the space in them is cut down to such an extent that a serious blood blockage could result. On the other hand if a person has wide arteries and cholesterol deposits pile up, there is still enough room for the blood to course through them freely.

Dr. Edgar Rentoul of Houston, Renfrewshire, England, in a special communication to *The Lancet* of December 12, 1953, was skirting around this field of speculation. He made the following points:

(1) "A few people are so genetically constituted that their coronary arteries are resistant to all adverse factors.

(2) "In the remainder the principal factors are of a simple mechanical nature: (a) the bigger the coronary arteries, the more room there is to have atheromatous plaques without disastrous results; (b) the faster the blood goes through the coronary arteries, the less likely it is that they will develop obstructions in their walls.

(3) "Assuming these statements to be correct, then the part played by exercise is clear. The more you exercise, the bigger your coronary arteries: the more you exercise, the faster the blood flows through them, the more difficult it is for an obstruction to develop on the walls.

(4) "I think that the exercise, to be really effective as a protector of the coronary arteries, must be fairly vigorous. The round of golf once a week is not much use."

Arteries can be narrow in any part of the body, but when this condition affects the coronary arteries there will be trouble ahead unless action is taken. There is another condition that could affect the heart arteries—the way they branch. It is something that is decided before birth and can never be changed. If the coronary arteries fork at a wide angle, the blood may form eddies and a gummy substance will be deposited that narrows down these blood vessels, and a fatal clot may form.

The great trunk artery, the aorta, can become so narrow that not even a match-stick can be inserted. It is a dangerous condition that leads to early death. Several operations were recently performed in which the aorta was cleaned out. The first thing the patient noticed after the operation was that his terribly cold feet became warm. A narrow aorta is inherited, usually.

Perhaps it's her spacious arteries that enable a woman to resist conditions that usually kill men. In June, 1957, Dr. A. M. Masters, speaking at the 106th annual meeting of the American Medical Association, stated that women have a consistently higher blood pressure than men, yet outlive them. They have more cholesterol in their arteries, yet die from this cause less frequently than men do.

Width of capillaries was found to be related to high blood pressure in a study of 100 patients whose cases were reported in *The Lancet* of June 29, 1957. In this study the width of the capillaries was examined in the nail-bed and in the conjunctiva of the eye, the conjunctiva being the membrane that lines the eyelids and covers the eyeball. Capillaries were classified as normal or very thin in the examination of patients.

In this study several facts were revealed. Where the capillaries were extremely thin, there was often a condition of proteinuria, or protein in the urine. "Very thin nail-bed capillaries were found in 48 of the 100 hypertensives (high blood pressure). In 100 control patients without hypertension very thin capillaries were found in the nail-bed in three patients and in the conjunctiva in three patients. . . . Severe conjunctival capillary thinning had a trend of association with proteinuria, changes in the fundus, and cerebral arteriopathy. Severe nail-bed capillary thinning was significantly correlated with severe conjunctival capillary thinning and severe heart disease."

The latter statement would seem to indicate that if the capillaries are thin in one part of the body, the condition is probably general throughout.

There is another test that may be significant. Dr. Hardin Jones of the University of California (*Time,* October 20, 1952) has worked out a way of finding out how much blood is flowing through the tissues. Says *Time,* "The more blood the younger the tissues, and hence the younger the body." The method is to measure the carbon dioxide given off by the muscles during exercise.

In testing 500 factory workers it was found that the average 18-year-old person had 25 cc. of blood passing through one liter of muscle per minute. At age 25 the average drops to 15 cc. By 35, it is down to 10 cc. But there seem to be enormous variations among seemingly healthy people. There is probably a wide variation in the width of arteries.

An interesting question about the width of arteries relates to mental power. Research should be performed to discover whether increasing the width of arteries in the brain can make a person think better. Is the width of brain arteries a factor in mental power? Would this answer the question as to why some children are infant prodigies? Is this the reason why some persons have photographic minds? Can we use this method to check on college entrance material? What a subject for research!

It is important for a person to determine if he was endowed with narrow blood vessels, for he can take measures to help himself. The body usually gives signals when the arteries are narrower than average. Persons with narrow arteries tend to have high blood pressure. Collateral circulation is apt to be poor, particularly in the lower limbs, manifesting itself in feet that get cold easily and sometimes turn numb.

The person with narrow arteries can help counteract this condition with vitamin E—one of the most important means to help the blood force itself through narrow arteries and restricted arterial areas. Rutin and vitamin C should also be taken because they build strength into the artery walls. Garlic pills should be taken because they are known to lower the blood pressure and dilate the blood vessels. He should take many other food supplements to help build general health into his body. And he should take plenty of exercise. In this way, it is possible that a health-conscious, narrow-arteried person might outlive a careless, wide-arteried one. It is the story of the hare and the tortoise.

All this good advice, of course, should not be restricted to those endowed with narrow arteries. For all people, diet is the key to a healthy heart and a vital system of circulation. In the second portion of this book, the "whys" and "hows" of healthy nutrition and its relation to heart disease will be examined at greater length.

Part Two: Diet and Circulatory Disorders

CHAPTER VI

Troublesome Fats

THERE IS general agreement among heart specialists that various fats circulating in the bloodstream lead to clogging of the blood vessels and result in arteriosclerosis and atherosclerosis. There is less agreement upon how to treat these diseases because there are five distinct types of fats which may be responsible.

Dr. Robert F. Zelis of the National Heart Institute, reporting to the American Heart Association on November 21, 1968, referred to studies done by his colleagues, Drs. Donald S. Frederickson and Robert I. Levy, which break the fats into the following types:

Type I: fat globules called "chylomicrons," which seldom result in heart attacks but create fatty deposits in the skin called "xanthomas."

Type II: lipoproteins, a low-density combination of fat with protein, including cholesterol, often associated with heart attacks.

Type III: denser, heavier lipoproteins composed of both cholesterol and the common fats called "triglycerides," also associated with heart attacks.

Type IV: fats of extremely low density, commonly found in overweight people and diabetics.

Type V: mixture of chylomicrons and tiny lipoproteins, often found in alcoholics and victims of inflammation of the pancreas.

Each type requires a different treatment, according to the NHI study, with Types I, IV and V responding best to a diet low in the specific kind of fat present. However, even when drugs were used to treat Types II and III, diets low in cholesterol and triglycerides were also used.

Treating the fats once they have become troublesome is only one aspect of the problem, however. The major controversy concerns how fat deposits came to be formed in the first place. As we shall see, this is a very complicated question, and it is impossible to single down on any one factor as *the* cause. Undoubtedly there are many causes.

In looking for culprits, however, the fats in our diet seem a logical place to begin. An obvious solution seems ready-made: if there is too much fat in the bloodstream, then eat less fat and the problem will go away. Cholesterol—one of the fats listed above in two categories—has received particular attention because it seems possible to relate a high cholesterol level in the blood with the advance of arteriosclerosis. So you would presume that cutting down on high cholesterol foods would automatically reduce the amount of blood cholesterol. Such easy answers, however, turn out to be uncertain, as will later be illustrated. No researcher anywhere in the world has been able to prove conclusively a cause-and-effect relationship between fat intake and fat deposits on the artery walls.

There is good reason, however, to believe that the amount of fats in a population's diet is related to the number of deaths from heart disease. Here are some samples of the many studies on this subject that have been made all over the world.

In the war years, when some of the European countries drastically cut their fat consumption, deaths from atherosclerosis declined considerably. For example, in France the death rate from coronary thrombosis from 1941 to 1945 was 20.6 per 100,000 of population. But after normal fat consumption was resumed, in the years from 1945 to 1949, the mortality rate from this disease went up to 25.5. The same condition held in Sweden, Finland, Norway and Italy. But in the United States, where there was no drop in fat consumption, there was a rise in the deaths from coronary diseases during the war years.

In Japan the diet consists of only about 8 percent fat against 40 percent for the United States.

In Italy it is only 20 percent. The heart disease mortality rate from aged 55 to 59 for men in the United States is four times that of Italy and ten times that of Japan.

Here is some interesting information from a bulletin issued by the University of Minnesota. (Vol. 24, No. 18. Feb. 20, 1953).

"A study was made in Madrid, Spain, 'on 55 poor men habitually on a low-fat diet (about 22 percent of calories from fats) and 57 prosperous professional men on a diet similar to that eaten by wealthy men in the United States. The poor men, moreover, were on a low-calorie diet. The prosperous professional men in Madrid are not much different from the Minnesota standards, but they are in great contrast to the poor Madrilenos, especially after 30 years of age.' The poor men have a much lower blood cholesterol content. 'There seems to be no doubt that coronary diseases are not common in Spain. This is agreed by the local doctors and is confirmed by a search through the hospitals. But it is also of interest that the leading fashionable physicians do not lack cases among their rich patients and tell of many relatives and colleagues who have died from occlusions.

" 'The data summarized here suggest an important chain of relations between the total fat content of the diet, the cholesterol concentration of the blood, the development of atherosclerosis, and the mortality from degenerative heart disease. The vital statistics data for Italy clearly fit this pattern.' "

A study was made in the Cape Peninsula of Africa of the fat in the diet and its relation to coronary artery diseases. It was done by B. Bronte-Stewart, M.D., of Cape Town, Ancel Keys of the University of Minnesota and several others, and was written up in *The Lancet* of November 26, 1955. A large group of men between the ages of 40 and 58 were studied, distributed between three racial groups—the Bantu, the Cape Negro and Europeans who resided in Cape Town. It was found that the Europeans consumed twice as much fat as the Bantus, with Cape Town Negroes about half way in between. In a study of 5,000 electrocardiograms it was found that coronary thrombosis was rare in Bantu—0.9 percent. In the Cape Negroes it was 6.8 percent and in the Europeans 13.54 percent, which to a certain extent followed the pattern of fat consumption of the three groups.

An experiment was performed by Lester M. Morrison, M.D., of Los Angeles, with 100 patients who had suffered a coronary thrombosis. (It is known that 90 percent of such cases are caused by atherosclerosis of the coronary arteries.) It was written up in the December 10, 1955, issue of the *Journal of the American Medical Association.* The people were divided into two groups—one in which no dietary fat-restriction was imposed, and the other which received not more than 20 to 25 grams of fat daily. After three years it was noted that of the group of 50 that had no fat restriction,

35 survived, 15 having died of coronary disease. But of the fat-restricted group, 43 survived, only 7 having died of coronary disease.

Upon checking eight years later, the restrictions having been continued, it was found that of the 50 unrestricted persons only 12 were still living, 38 having died of coronary disease. But of the fat-restricted group, 28 were still living, only 22 having died of coronary disease.

Despite such studies, however, there are many puzzling contradictions in the evidence. An example can be found in a study by A. S. Loginov, published in the Russian heart journal, *Kardiologiya* (2, 1, 1962). Drawing on statistics concerned with Ethiopia, the study showed that changes in diet in that North African country did affect the blood serum level of cholesterol, but that regardless of serum level Ethiopia had practically no heart disease.

Other studies have shown that while many victims of atherosclerosis and ischemic heart disease have high levels of serum cholesterol, there are others who do not. And equally puzzling has been the fact that very large portions of our population show high serum cholesterol on testing, yet never develop heart or circulatory diseases.

A. M. Cohen reported in the *American Heart Journal* (65, 291, 1963) that Jews living in Yemen eat very high fat diets yet have little heart disease. whereas those of the same national strain who have migrated to Israel where they eat a more "civilized" and less primitive diet, show the same tendency to contract atherosclerosis as is noticeable in Western Europe and the United States.

To begin to understand the complicated problem, it is important to distinguish between two different types of fats—those that are saturated and those that are unsaturated.

Saturated and Unsaturated Fats

Fatty substances are made up of various atoms of carbon, hydrogen and oxygen, linked together like chains. Some are long, meaning they have many atoms linked together; others are short. Some kinds of fats have open links, you might say, where other atoms can be attached to them. These are called the "unsaturated fatty acids." By "unsaturated" we mean that these open links in the chain are there, ready to be filled or "saturated" with an atom of some other substance.

Linolenic, linoleic and arachidonic acids are just such "unsaturated" fatty acids. That is why they are so extremely valuable to good health. They have open links in their chain of atoms and they are ready, willing and able to combine with other substances in the big chemical laboratory that is the body. So they take part in all kinds of different things that go on. They can combine with other parts of food; they can help to carry these other parts of food through the miles of blood vessels, and they are used in building cell structure. They can do all this because—and only because—the open links in their chains of atoms invite other substances to join with them in various chemical combinations.

Well and good, you may say, so all we have to do is eat plenty of fat and we'll get enough unsaturated fatty acids to be healthful. Of course it's not that simple. First of all, certain things can happen to these *unsaturated* fatty acids that change them to *saturated* fatty acids before we eat them. In this case, the open chains have already been filled with some other substance and there is no chance that this kind of fat can take the active part it should take in the body's laboratory.

When oxygen is combined with the unsaturated fatty acids, an atom of oxygen moves into the empty link and joins itself chemically with the other atoms. The fat becomes rancid. When hydrogen is added, it moves into the empty link, joins itself to the other atoms and we have what is known as "hydrogenated fat"—a thick, almost solid, substance like lard. In both cases, of course, since the empty links have been filled, the fat can no longer fulfill its duties inside the body, because it is now "saturated"—there is no place for body substances to join with it and help in the work of the body.

Naturally nobody ever purposely makes fats rancid, for the taste is unpleasant and rancid fat in the diet is responsible for the destruction of fat-soluble vitamins. So rancid fats should be carefully avoided. Natural fats in their natural state, such as those in sunflower seeds, for instance, carry along with them substances called anti-oxidants which prevent oxygen from turning the fat rancid. But in many of the processes to which our table and cooking oils are subjected today, the anti-oxidants are destroyed.

Margarine is hydrogenated—most of the unsaturated fatty acids in it are destroyed. Cooking fats—the solid white ones like Crisco—have been hydrogenated. Processed cheeses are hydrogenated and so is peanut butter. This process of adding hydrogen to so many otherwise healthful foods may eventually have to bear the responsibility for a lot of our present-day ills.

People who depend on processed foods for their unsaturated fatty acids are just not going to get them. And people who are told by their doctors to eat a fat-free diet are not going to get them. People who eat diets high in animal fats are not going to get them, for they are most abundant in vegetable and cereal fats, and not at all plentiful in animal fats, such as butter, eggs, milk and meat fats.

An experiment with laboratory rats led British Dr. Hugh M. Sinclair and his associate, Dr. V. Basnayake, to the theory that cholesterol deposits on the walls of our arteries may result from too much *saturated* fat in our diets and too little *unsaturated* fat. According to their article in *The Lancet*, April 17, 1956, they fed the rats on a diet that contained no fats at all, but which was a good diet in other respects. What did they find? Large cholesterol deposits in the arteries of the animals. The longer the diet went on, the more cholesterol accumulated.

Now we are told that cholesterol deposits come from too much fat in the diet. How then could these rats, who were getting no fat at all, develop cholesterol deposits? Dr. Sinclair tells us that their bodies were manufacturing it—and we know that cholesterol is indeed manufactured in our bodies as well as coming from our food. And the reason that it accumulated had to be simply that a fat-free diet prevented the rats from getting any of the unsaturated fatty acids, which must be present in order to keep the cholesterol from depositing where it is not wanted.

It is impossible for us to imagine a daily diet for human beings entirely free from fat, so there is little danger that we may have the same experience the rats had. But as Dr. Sinclair goes on to say, the more cholesterol and the more *saturated* fat you have in your diet the more *unsaturated* fat you need, if you want to avoid cholesterol deposits. Then, too, if you have enough pyridoxine, the B vitamin, in your diet, you are likely to avoid trouble, for this vitamin can help out when the important fatty acids are not there.

Animal and vegetable fats in our diets have become increasingly oxidized and deprived of E. F. A. (Essential Fatty Acids) because of modern food processing. Vegetable oils, in many cases rich in E.

F. A., are hardened by hydrogenation; margarine and shortenings are produced by hydrogenation of cottonseed and soybean oil, some peanut-oil and certain other oils; during this hydrogenation much of the E. F. A. is destroyed and unnatural *trans* fatty acids are formed not only during hydrogenation but also during the practice of deep-frying.

How else do we lose these important food elements? Well, they occur in the germ of cereals which our food processors carefully remove and discard when they make white flour and packaged cereals. In addition, the flour "improvers," the bleaches, and many other chemicals that go into baked goods these days undoubtedly have some destructive action on the fatty acids. We have no idea how extensive this may be. In addition, when foods are refined, pyridoxine, that might get in a few good licks to help the situation, is also removed and discarded.

Dr. B. Bronte-Stewart and his associates in South Africa, whose work we cited earlier, were one of the pioneer research groups studying saturated vs. unsaturated fats in the diet. Commenting on their findings, *Science News Letter* for April 29, 1956, said: "The new and hopeful approach to stopping the nation's greatest disease killer, atherosclerosis, and consequent heart disease, results from a discovery by a team of South African scientists at the University of Cape Town.

"Dr. Bronte-Stewart and his group were able to separate from sunflower seed oil a highly unsaturated fatty acid and a saturated fatty acid fraction. They fed these to a patient whose blood cholesterol had been raised by adding cholesterol to his basic diet.

"When the unsaturated fraction was fed, the blood cholesterol promptly fell, even though the patient went on getting extra cholesterol in his diet. When the saturated fraction was fed, the cholesterol in his blood rose.

"They also point out that other factors besides fat in the diet may play a role in hardening of the arteries in some cases. Lack of physical exercise, occupational tensions, emotional states and perhaps also heavy smoking are among such factors."

An article in *The Lancet* of April 28, 1956, commenting on the experiments of Bronte-Stewart and his group, says "Food fats and oils thus seem to fall into two classes whose effects on plasma lipids (fats) are antagonistic to each other. If these results are substantiated, coronary artery disease becomes in part a preventable disorder—but at the cost of a complete revolution in our present-day dietary habits. The hydrogenation plants of our modern food industry may turn out to have contributed to the causation of a major disease."

Many other studies corroborate the conclusion that there is an important difference between the unsaturated fats and the saturated fats—and that the latter is the one to avoid in your diet.

In experiments done at the Highland Alameda County Hospital at Oakland, California, as reported in the *Journal of Clinical Nutrition* for March, 1953, it was found that, "patients maintained on chemically constant diets containing very large amounts of fat of vegetable origin, without exception have striking falls in plasma cholesterol."

A research team from Harvard and investigators in the Federal Medical Department of Nigeria found that the Nigerians consume large quantities of vegetable fats but have considerably lower blood cholesterol levels than Americans. (*British Medical Journal,* 2, 1008, 1955.) These are but two examples of a large body of similar scientific findings.

In review, which fats should you avoid and which should you feel safe in eating if you want to prevent hardening of the arteries and heart disorders?

Animal fats in general are high in cholesterol and low in unsaturated fatty acids—fatty meats, lard, milk, butter and cheese should be eliminated or greatly curtailed in your diet. Vegetable fats should predominate. These should *not* include margarine or any of the hydrogenated fats—the solid ones generally used for shortenings, processed cheeses, or commercial hydrogenated peanut butter. Salad oils (vegetable oils in liquid state) are good food, high in unsaturated fatty acids. Natural whole foods like nuts, sunflower seeds, wheat germ, avocados, etc., are the best source of all. The health food supplement, lecithin, is valuable chiefly for its unsaturated fatty acid content. Wheat germ oil and fish liver oil are rich in unsaturated fatty acids.

CHAPTER VII

How Carbohydrates Cause Problems

FAT IN THE DIET—whether saturated or unsaturated—is by no means the only factor affecting the fat level in our blood. Carbohydrates—foods high in sugar and starch—also play a role. Experiments have shown that fat intake can actually be reduced drastically and still the blood fat level will rise if the person is on a diet of carbohydrate-rich foods.

A researcher at the Rockefeller Institute, Dr. Edward H. Ahrens, found that a diet rich in carbohydrates and low in fats tended to raise the level of fats in the blood. The *New York Times* for May 4, 1961, reported that Dr. Ahrens spent nine years testing various diets on volunteers. Thirteen of those tested developed the highest levels of blood fat *on the diet that contained no fat at all!*

The lowest blood fat levels were noted on a diet that contained 70 percent fat. It did not seem to make much difference whether the fats in the diet were saturated or unsaturated.

The diets used in the experiments were the exaggerated kinds used in many experiments where the researcher wants to emphasize greatly one aspect of what he is investigating, so that there can be no possible doubt as to what his results mean. One of the diets eaten consisted of 85 percent carbohydrate, 15 percent protein and no fat at all. Another consisted of only 15 percent carbohydrate, 15 percent protein and 70 percent fat. It is most unlikely that any of us would be eating such diets since they are so far removed from the kind of food one gets in everyday meals, but they certainly show that when Dr. Ahrens says a certain thing about a diet high in carbohydrates, he indeed has tested just such a diet.

In 1958 John W. Gofman, Alex V. Nichols and E. Virginia Dobbin, of the University of California, wrote a fine book, *Dietary Prevention and Treatment of Heart Disease* (G. P. Putnam's Sons) in which they talked extensively about the possible role of carbohydrates, along with fats, in forming unwanted fatty deposits on artery walls.

In answering the question "How is it that dietary intake of carbohydrates, a foodstuff class which is wholly different from fat, has the ability to raise the amount of certain fat-like materials in the blood?" these authors say, "The final answer to this question is not available. We know that the effect does occur. . . . One . . . possibility is that when the person is taking in a great deal of carbohydrates, and thus making sugar available in fair quantities, the metabolism of the body may use the sugar preferentially as a fuel for energy. Thus the rate at which certain fat-like materials are used for energy purposes may be slowed down, allowing a build-up in the amount of these fat-like materials in the bloodstream. This, of course, is a deleterious result from the point of view of arterial thickening since it is the amount of the fat-like substances *of the blood* which is important!"

The book written by these investigators contains valuable charts giving the carbohydrate content of foods, showing those containing 0-9 percent carbohydrates, those containing 10-19 percent carbohydrates and those containing 20 percent and more carbohydrates, also charts showing the saturated and unsaturated fats in various foods.

The 20 percent and more carbohydrate foods are cereals, bakery products, desserts and prepared, sugared or dried fruits, almost exclusively. Those below 20 percent carbohydrates are the other fresh fruits and vegetables. Saturated fats occur in greatest quantity in processed foods, desserts and those in which lard, butter, milk or hydrogenated shortenings have been used. Unsaturated fats occur in fruits and vegetables, whole grains and seeds, and vegetable and cereal oils.

Another worker in the field is Benjamin P. Sandler, M.D., of Veterans Hospital, Oteen, North Carolina. Dr. Sandler's book, *How to Prevent Heart Attacks* (published by Lee Foundation, Milwaukee, Wisconsin), discussed in great detail the relation of blood sugar levels to heart pain and attacks. The author states, "The patient with heart pain experiences all of the ill effects of reduced oxygen inhalation whenever the blood sugar level is abnormally reduced. Hypoglycemia (low blood sugar) absolute or relative, means reduced oxygen consumption by all cells that require sugar for energy purposes. The heart muscle suffers an oxygen lack of varying degree every time the blood sugar falls at an abnormally rapid rate."

What causes the blood sugar to fall? Habitual consumption of too much carbohydrate-rich food in relation to the amount of protein and fat consumed. So Dr. Sandler is saying in another way, just what Dr. Gofman and his associates and Dr. Ahrens are saying—if you would be free from heart and artery trouble, shun the carbohydrate-rich foods. They are real troublemakers.

Of the carbohydrates, sugar is so deeply implicated as a contributor to heart and artery disease that it will be discussed at length in a separate chapter.

The basis of Dr. Sandler's recommended diet for preventing heart trouble is protein. All foods of animal origin he says may be eaten in unlimited quantities, including eggs and milk. Any food containing sugar is forbidden—that is, all desserts, soft drinks, jams, pastries, ice cream and so forth. The starchy foods are to be eaten in reduced quantities: all foods of the spaghetti-noodle variety, beans and potatoes. Fruits with high-sugar contents should be eaten in limited quantities. All other fruits and vegetables may be eaten in unlimited quantities. Dr. Sandler does not forbid or limit fats. Nor does he make a distinction among the different kinds of carbohydrates, although the carbohydrates in fresh fruits—bananas, for instance—have a quite different effect from those in cereals, especially the refined cereals.

In France, an article in *Archives des Malaises du Coeur* for March, 1960, by E. Hoareau and G. Delanoe, tells of their studies of 738 heart patients in Morocco. Of these, 111 had hardening of the arteries. Comparing their observations with those of other French researchers, they found that heart diseases due to hardening of the arteries were four times more frequent in Morocco than in Paris. Figures on heart diseases due to hardening of the arteries did not run parallel to those for cholesterol, seeming to indicate that these heart patients in Morocco had normal levels of cholesterol.

The French researchers believe that a deficiency in protein food plays a major part in the occurrence of heart conditions due to hardening of the arteries. Moroccans do not have enough protein in their diets, especially protein of animal origin like meat and eggs. The French scientists believe also that an excess of calories from white sugar and white flour products might have the effect of causing deposits on the artery walls, resulting in artery hardening.

One might decide that such could not be the case in America where there is plenty of animal protein available. But there are infallible statistics showing that about one-half of the calories of the American diet derive from white sugar and white flour products.

Many surveys have been done showing that individual diets may be seriously lacking in animal protein and very high in refined carbohydrates. Every survey we have seen which dealt with the diet of teenagers testifies eloquently to the serious deficiencies of most teenage diets. Cake, Cokes, white bread, candy, all easily available and inexpensive, form far too large a part of the diet of young folks. Among older people, starchy and sweet foods are popular because they are easy to prepare, tasty and soft.

We think there is a valuable lesson to be learned from all the information we have presented above, indicating that starches and sweets are certainly one of the evils, if not the main evil, in hardening of the arteries and heart disease. The lesson is that, if one automatically eliminates the refined sugars and starches from his meals, he will have substituted for them lots of protein foods of animal origin—meat, fish, poultry, eggs. He will be eating plenty of fresh fruits, vegetables and nuts. Just to be on the safe side, he will also go easy on animal fats like butter, and will shun entirely the processed fats like margarine and the solid white shortenings.

Taking brewer's yeast and/or desiccated liver for additional protein and B vitamins, as well as other food supplements for vitamins and minerals, he should be as free from fear of heart disease as anyone can be in modern times.

CHAPTER VIII

What Sugar Does to the Circulatory System

NEARLY two million people will die in the United States this year, according to estimates based on figures from the National Office of Vital Statistics. More than half of those, a full million, will die as a result of arteriosclerosis and hypertension. Of this unfortunate million, there is reason to believe, at least half will have developed atherosclerosis, the condition leading to their deaths, because of too much sugar in their diets.

Evidence is mounting that sugar in the diet is perhaps the primary villain in causing death from heart and circulatory disease. A pioneer advocate of this theory is the famous British nutritionist, Professor John Yudkin, of the University of London, whose profound knowledge leaves him appalled at what modern civilization is doing to its citizens.

Many scientists, some of whose work will be reported later on in this chapter, now support Professor Yudkin's findings. But the average doctor to whom you take your problems is likely to ignore this aspect of diet control, since so much emphasis has always been laid on fat intake.

In the July 4, 1964, issue of *The Lancet,* Professor Yudkin pointed out his reasons for believing that the medical profession is on the wrong track when it tries to connect heart disease only with the amount of fat consumed in the diet.

Quoting studies made by the Food and Agriculture Organization of the United Nations, Professor Yudkin points out that while it is true that fat consumption increases as countries and their populations grow wealthier, sugar consumption increases with it and at an even faster rate. "Intakes of fat and sugar . . . not only rise by the same high factor of about four-fold from the poorest group of countries to the wealthiest group but are almost exactly the same in absolute quantities. (However) the relative constancy of carbohydrate intake with increase in income hides an increase in sugar intake, which almost exactly matches the fall in other carbohydrates, mostly starch."

In other words, the consumption of fat and of carbohydrate increase at just about the same rate with an increase in the means to buy them. However, within the carbohydrate group the consumption of starches is reduced and the consumption of sugars increased. This indicates, as shown by Dr.

Yudkin in a chart derived from statistics from 41 countries, that of all foods, it is sugar that has the fastest increasing rate of consumption in the wealthier countries where the rate of deaths by heart disease keeps increasing at an equally fast rate. And it is just as reasonable to suppose that the increase in heart disease is due to the increased intake of sugar as it is to suppose it is because of more fat in the diet.

The reason why most investigators have concentrated on the fat is primarily because the sugar intake is more masked. Sugar is added to most processed foods today, from a can of tomatoes to a package of frozen chicken a la king, because it adds palatability to the sterilized and flavorless messes today's food manufacturers sell for popular consumption. Thus it is very hard to make an estimate of how much sugar we are actually consuming, whereas the intake of fat is far more obvious.

Your doctor might be very surprised to learn that the average per capita consumption of sugar in this country is more than half a pound a day. He knows that even a quarter pound a day is far, far too much, and given any idea of how high a patient's sugar consumption may be, he would probably try to reduce it. But even with sincere and strenuous efforts, it would be virtually impossible for the average person eating an average diet of processed foods to reduce his sugar consumption to a proper level. Even if he eliminates all sweet drinks and desserts, there remain fantastic quantities of the sweet poison in practically every food that has had anything to do with the factory before reaching the consumer. Dr. Yudkin estimates that a full 50 percent of the sugar consumption of the average individual, which is to say roughly a quarter pound a day, is derived from sugar added in food processing—sugar you do not even know you are eating.

Nevertheless, that leaves the other 50 percent which you yourself add to your diet if you are so ill-advised as to be a user of refined sugar. And the fact that some people use sugar without any heed of consequences while others attempt to eliminate sugar as much as they possibly can, leaves scope for tremendous variation in the individual consumption of sugar. If the per capita figure is half a pound a day, we can say with confidence that there are many people who eat a quarter pound or less of sugar daily, and many others who may consume a pound or more every day of their lives.

It is precisely on this question of individual variation that the cholesterol theory of the causation of heart disease is at its weakest. Statistically, analyzing a large group of people or an entire population, you can show that as cholesterol in the diet increases, so does heart disease. But when it comes to examining the individuals who actually suffer from heart disease, it has proven impossible to pin down a definite relationship.

Just such a definite relationship, however, has been shown between sugar and heart disease in a study Dr. Yudkin made of two groups of London Hospital patients. The first group consisted of those who had been admitted to the hospital for either a recent heart attack or an atherosclerotic condition. The second group consisted of those admitted for accidental injuries who, except for the accidents they had suffered, could be said to be in good health and were not known to have any kind of difficulties concerning the heart or circulatory system. The second group was to be studied as a control, to be contrasted with group one.

What Dr. Yudkin found was that *without exception* the hospital patients with arterial disease were consuming substantially more sugar than those in the control group. On the average they were consuming twice as much. Even more remarkable as a confirmation, it was found that "in patients with peripheral arterial disease, more detailed analysis suggests that the degree of atherosclerosis was proportional to the amount of dietary sugar." In other words, it was possible to do in this single study what could not be done in ten years of studying the possible relationship between fat consumption and atherosclerosis. It was possible to show statistically that not only is the atherosclerotic a heavy user of sugar, but the more sugar he uses the worse is his atherosclerotic condition.

Most remarkable of all, it was found so uniformly and without exception that the sufferer from atherosclerosis is a user of unusually large amounts of sugar, that even a small number of samples produced a statistically significant correlation.

Here's how that works. Suppose you want to find out whether there is a relationship between two elements—let's say, wearing brown shoes and being a good walker. You take a hundred good walkers and see how many of them wear brown shoes. If you find that 60 wear brown shoes and 40 wear black, this may or may not be of some significance. You then have to examine a thousand good walkers or ten thousand or a hundred thousand until you reach a point where it becomes mathematically inescapable that the two factors either are or are not related. But if among your randomly selected 100 good walkers, you find that every single one of them wears brown shoes, then you know immediately that there is a significant relationship. It can no longer be the result of sheer coincidence or accident.

And it is for precisely this same reason that Professor Yudkin's study, even though a small one, is a highly significant one. The chance that the relationship he has shown between high sugar consumption and atherosclerosis could occur accidentally is computed to be less than one in two thousand. This brings it very close to certainty that eating large amounts of sugar is a prime cause of the disease that kills more of us than any other and is far and away responsible for more deaths in middle age than is any other.

Our ancestors a hundred years ago ate perhaps two pounds of sugar a year. This is practically no sugar at all, yet they could work harder for longer hours, think loftier and clearer thoughts, raise larger families and in every way demonstrate very high energy levels. You don't need sugar for energy. It is nothing but sweet poison that begins attacking a person's teeth the moment it enters the mouth and never stops attacking somewhere as long as it remains in the system.

They say the price of sugar is rising. If we could get it free, the price would still be too high.

A number of studies now back up Dr. Yudkin's findings. In 1965, three doctors from Czechoslovakia wrote to *The Lancet* saying they too have observed that excess consumption of sugar is associated with increasing heart disease. Using food consumption data from the ten regions of Czechoslovakia, they found that people in the districts with highest sugar use had the most heart disease. Fat consumption was not as closely related to mortality from cardiovascular disease. Although they recommend "cutting down the high consumption of sugar so usual in industrial countries," they caution against drawing definite conclusions from the data now available.

The June, 1965, issue of the *Annals of Internal Medicine* contains four reports of studies linking sugar to heart attack. In one, a group of Michigan researchers observed the whole population (9,500) of the Michigan community of Tecumseh and found that blood sugar levels were significantly related to hardening of the arteries. A Philadelphia project reported in the same issue found a link between sugar in the diet and blood triglycerides, a type of fat which some authorities believe is as troublesome as cholesterol.

Later that same year it was announced that routine diabetic screening tests may someday be used to help detect the early symptoms of heart disease. The possibility was suggested in an editorial in the September 18, 1965, issue of *The Lancet.* Referring to the tests as valuable tools in spotting unrecognized high blood sugar levels in the population, the journal pointed out that there is growing evidence that these high sugar levels may also be the first signs of arterial disease. "We may thus be approaching a time when the early detection of asymptomatic high blood-sugar in the population at large will be an important preliminary to measures for its correction in order to reduce the increasing toll of cardiovascular disease," the editorial concludes.

Probably basis for *The Lancet's* position on the sugar and heart disease link was a study reported in an earlier issue of the journal showing that even minor elevations of blood sugar may possibly carry an increased risk of heart disease. Dr. Harry Keen of Guys Hospital in London and five colleagues surveyed the symptoms of heart disease among three groups of people—those found to have a high blood sugar level (diabetes), those with moderately raised blood sugar, and a third group with normal sugar levels. Writing in the September 11, 1965, issue of *The Lancet,* the researchers pointed out that the prevalence of the symptoms of arterial disease was lowest in the control group, intermediate in the border line group and highest in the diabetics. "We conclude that the association between these various manifestations of arterial disease and the level of glucose tolerance is real, and that this conclusion holds even at those levels of blood sugar at which a diagnosis of diabetes is considered doubtful," Dr. Keen and his associates pointed out.

Other researchers in almost every corner of the world are also accumulating solid evidence that an excessive intake of sugar is a primary cause of the modern epidemic of heart disease. A California physician warned individuals to "take a close look at the sugar bowl" if they intend to avoid heart attacks. Dr. Clifford Anderson, the popular medical commentator, said sugar builds up fatty tissue on the inside of coronary arteries which might clot and cause a heart attack. Another study showed that a group of heart attack victims had been taking about 4.5 ounces of sugar a day while a control group of healthy men ate only 2.75 ounces of sugar, Dr. Anderson said. Criticizing the recent trend toward prepared pre-sweetened cereals, Dr. Anderson called it a "shocking thing that young people should be brought up on this stuff."

Simple vs. Complex Carbohydrates

Writing in the November, 1965, issue of the *American Journal of Clinical Nutrition,* Drs. Robert E. Hodges and W. A. Krehl of the University of Iowa College of Medicine suggested that diets rich in refined white sugar and other simple carbohydrates may play an important role in elevating cholesterol and other fats in the blood. Basis for that conclusion is a series of dietary studies of five groups of volunteers showing that high intakes of refined sugar triggered rises in cholesterol levels despite the fact that the levels of saturated fatty acids in the diets remained constant throughout the studies. "The results of the experiments . . . indicate that a high intake of simple sugars is accompanied by an increase in the concentration of cholesterol and other fats in the blood," Drs. Hodges and Krehl reported.

However, the Iowa researchers also discovered that when the simple sugars were replaced by complex carbohydrates (potatoes, cereals and bread), cholesterol and triglyceride levels actually fell. Explaining their study further, the scientists said that the experiments were designed to compare the effects of feeding diets equal in caloric value and containing the same percentage of proteins, carbohydrates and fats, but in which the source of carbohydrates was changed from sugar to complex carbohydrates. "Initially, the cholesterol level rose when sugar was fed, declined slightly when starch (complex carbohydrate) was fed, rose again when sugar was fed and fell again when starch was fed," Drs. Hodges and Krehl explained. According to the researchers, a similar pattern was observed in each of the patient groups taking part in the study. "Experiments in man suggest that the concentration of cholesterol and lipids (fats) in the blood can be altered by interchanging complex carbohydrates and sugar in the diet," they concluded.

The Iowa physicians also reported two unexpected findings resulting from their study. Referring to the fact that the subjects were fed meals nearly equal in size, the researchers concluded that "feeding three equal meals daily rather than the customary pattern of unequal meals resulted in lower levels of cholesterol and glycerides in the blood." Even more important is the discovery that the subjects complained of being hungry when the simple sugars were served and of being "stuffed" when they received the complex carbohydrates. "Thus, it would seem that an increase in complex carbohydrates may serve a dual purpose in providing greater satiety as well as in lessening serum lipids," Drs. Hodges and Krehl explained.

Backing up the results obtained in their own study, the University of Iowa scientists cited a long list of both animal and human studies indicating that sugar may be involved in the heart disease problem. Much attention is given to the studies of Professor Yudkin. The researchers also point to the work of Dr. Ancel Keys who fed men diets differing in the proportion of carbohydrates supplied from the various food sources. When sucrose and simple carbohydrates were replaced by complex carbohydrates derived from fruits, vegetables, legumes and green, leafy vegetables, serum cholesterol levels decreased, Drs. Hodges and Krehl concluded from the Keys study.

One of the most important studies was published in the November, 1967, *American Journal of Clinical Nutrition* by these same authors, Drs. Krehl and Hodges, and two associates, Alfredo Lopez-S. and Eleanor I. Good. After reviewing the dietary habits and heart disease death rates of people living in western countries, this group of expert nutritionists has confirmed that the type of carbohydrate eaten is basic in the development of atherosclerotic heart disease. The overall amount of carbohydrates has changed little in recent years, they point out, but there has been a significant switch away from consumption of complex carbohydrates—the starches of such foods as cereals, potatoes and vegetables—and an increase in the intake of simple carbohydrates such as refined sugar and the foods that contain it like syrups and sweets.

In the new book *Diet and Disease* by Drs. Cheraskin, Ringsdorf and Clark of the University of Alabama (Rodale Press, 1968), the even more positive conclusion is drawn that the eating in any quantity of simple carbohydrates such as refined sugar increased the blood cholesterol level significantly, while the eating of complex carbohydrates such as potatoes actually *reduced* the amount of cholesterol in the blood.

All would seem to lead to the conclusion that anyone troubled with a high level of blood cholesterol could not do better for himself than immediately to eliminate all sugar from his diet.

That is also the theme of the book, *How to Prevent Heart Attacks*, by Benjamin P. Sandler, M.D., whom we quoted earlier. Dr. Sandler believes that low sugar in the blood is the cause of heart disease.

How does a high sugar diet lead to a low level of sugar in the blood? When one ingests sugar, or starch that turns to sugar, insulin is secreted in the pancreatic gland in order to prevent it from raising the level of sugar in the blood. The function of the insulin is to keep the sugar down. But if too much insulin is secreted as occurs when large amounts of sugar are ingested, then the sugar in the blood declines considerably. The liver, certain glands and part of the nervous system also enter into the process, but it is the insulin directly that lowers the blood sugar. One of the clues that convinced Dr. Sandler of the dangers of carbohydrates and sugar to heart cases was the fact that in diabetics—whose ability to produce insulin is impaired—heart disease is more serious, occurs at an earlier age, and is more common.

In order to understand how this theory works

we must know the effect of sugar on the heart's action. "The heart muscle is made up of innumerable muscle cells," says Dr. Sandler. "Like all muscle tissue, it needs certain nutrients to perform its work of contraction and relaxation. The chief nutrients are sugar and oxygen, both of which are brought to the muscle by the blood. . . . In the muscle cells, the sugar and oxygen react chemically to yield the necessary energy needed for the work of contraction. . . . Among the many varied and complicated chemical reactions that occur during (heart) muscle contraction, is the production of lactic acid. . . . Under certain conditions, lactic acid may accumulate in abnormal quantities in a muscle, including the heart, and it is believed that this accumulation of lactic acid along with a few other acid metabolites produced during muscle contraction is responsible for the heart pain. One of the conditions that may cause this abnormal accumulation of metabolites is the . . . abnormally low sugar utilization by the heart muscle. . . . Any significant interference with the supply of sugar or oxygen will embarrass heart action, and the degree of interference will determine the degree of embarrassment—from a mild fleeting chest pain to the severe crushing pain of the fatal heart attack."

But it isn't merely the low blood sugar that does the harm. Dr. Sandler has found from experience that it is the violent fluctuations in the blood sugar that create trouble. Eating a meal rich in carbohydrates will do that because first it raises the blood sugar, then it lowers it. "The rapid rate of change in the downward direction results in a severe environmental change for the heart muscle to which it fails to accommodate readily and so the muscle is embarrassed and the symptoms of pain are felt by the patient."

In addition to sugar, as has already been said, oxygen is important to the healthful operation of the heart muscle. Quoting Dr. Sandler, "It has been shown that a cell utilizes oxygen in proportion as it utilizes sugar. But oxygen is useful to the cell only if there is some fuel to burn (oxidize) for the production of energy. The blood may be normally saturated with oxygen but if the blood sugar level is half of what it should be, the body will consume less than normal oxygen. . . . It has been accepted by many that the immediate cause of heart pain is an acute oxygen lack on the part of the heart muscle."

The proof of the pudding is in the eating, says Dr. Sandler, because the low carbohydrate diet he devised has been successful in many cases in giving relief from attacks of heart pain, and in preventing their occurrence.

The American Medical Association recognized the importance of carbohydrate nutrition and metabolism to coronary heart disease control in an editorial in the September 25, 1967, issue of its *Journal.*

Three main points were made:

1. A single diet plan won't suffice to provide best coronary disease prevention in all people. However, it was pointed out that 90 percent of the experimental subjects observed by Dr. P. T. Kuo, a leading investigator of the carbohydrate-heart link, reacted very favorably to a diet low in simple carbohydrates and high in complex carbohydrates. *The Journal of the American Medical Association* article noted that "Kuo's data indicate that sensitivity to simple carbohydrate is widespread among both healthy and atherosclerotic populations in America."

2. Although there are still gaps in our present knowledge, the AMA noted that triglycerides and carbohydrate metabolism have a fundamental role as diet factors involved in the cause of coronary disease.

3. It is now up to physicians to find out which of their patients in the high-risk coronary disease group react unfavorably to a high fat diet, which are sensitive to carbohydrates of the wrong sort, and which people may be being led to increased heart risk by both of those dietary factors.

CHAPTER IX

The Effects of Hard Water and Trace Minerals

ALTHOUGH THERE IS general agreement among specialists of the need for various minerals in human nutrition, the controversy over hard versus soft water has been raging for several decades. Obviously, hard water (water with a high calcium and magnesium content) is more inconvenient to work with than soft water because the latter forms suds easier.

Water softeners guarantee quick, thick suds, true, but the most commonly used means of water softening transfers two parts of sodium to the softened water for every part of calcium or magnesium removed. The danger of the added sodium to health far outweighs the convenience factors that may be gained.

A London Hospital Medical College team, Drs. J. N. Norris, M. D. Crawford and J. A. Heady, found, according to a report in the *New York Times* (May 7, 1961): "The softer the water supply in the country boroughs of England, the higher the death rate from cardiovascular disease. What this means is not at present clear, and further investigation is indicated."

The team agreed that the main problem was to decide whether there was a cause-and-effect relationship between heart disease and soft water. They were not sure if the minerals in the hard water actually had some preservative effect, or if soft water, either natural or treated, carries harmful trace elements which have an adverse effect on the heart. Whatever the reason, it is obvious that to trade hard water for soft is to invite increased likelihood of heart disease. Either something in hard water protects against heart ailments, or something in soft water promotes them, according to these scientists.

Their work, it turned out, was a British version of work done in the United States by Dr. Henry Schroeder of Dartmouth Medical School, and reported in the *Journal of the American Medical Association* (April 23, 1960). Dr. Schroeder found that, in general, the watershed areas of the Mississippi, Missouri and Ohio Rivers had hard water and lower death rates and that the Altantic and Pacific Coast states had softer water and higher death rates. Dr. Schroeder found the connection between cardiovascular disease and soft water to be significant, though not proved. "It seems to me to be fairly well established—not that soft water is the cause of cardiovascular disease, but that it has some influence on death rates."

The salt content of soft water is an important consideration in determining its relationship to the incidence of heart disease. Salt-free diets are very often recommended by doctors treating patients for heart disease, dropsy and circulatory disturbances. That is because salt increases the volume of the blood through water retention and therefore raises the blood pressure.

Dr. Frederick Allen introduced the low salt diet for high blood pressure to this country, and was quoted in the *Journal of the American Medical Association,* June 4, 1949, as saying: "My conclusion, based on unique experience in several thousand cases during 28 years, is that saltless diets, especially when begun reasonably early, can specifically arrest progressiveness, prevent complications and thus provide the first real control of deaths from hypertension."

Dr. Leo A. Saperstein of the University of Southern California, wrote in the *Proceedings of the Society of Experimental and Biological Medicine* (73: 82-85) of his experiments which showed that feeding salt to rats induced high blood pressure, and enlarged their hearts and kidneys. When water picks up salt through the softening process, its potential harm for persons suffering from hypertension is obvious. "During the fall of 1960 a water softener using zeolite as an absorbent was installed in the local Dinsmore Union Hospital, all the water used in the hospital being routed through the softener," reported Dr. David J. Bryant in the *Canadian Medical Association Journal,* February 25, 1961. Dr. Bryant continues that diuretic drugs such as hydrochlorothiazide, "used in the treatment of hypertension and edema of congestive heart failure, etc., were suddenly found to have little or no expected effect . . . it was recognized that the water softener was converting the water used in the hospital for every purpose into a mild saline solution, and as a result had all of our hospital patients on a fairly high sodium diet."

Dr. Schroeder was consulted on a question printed in Questions and Answers in the *Journal of the American Medical Association,* May 20, 1961. A Jacksonville, Florida, doctor wanted to know if a water softener is likely to put sufficient sodium in the water for it to be harmful to a patient on a low sodium diet. Dr. Schroeder said first that the amount of sodium put into the water would vary with the hardness of the water "and the present efficiency of the softener." (The efficiency varies with the amount of time the softener is in use.) He also noted that the amount of sodium which is naturally present in the local water supply is different in different places. Then, too, some municipalities soften hard water at the water treatment plants, with zeolite soda lime. "which can add a large amount of sodium."

Dr. Schroeder gives, as an indication of the high

sodium content possible in the water we take from the tap, the reading for the water supply at Sarasota, Florida (530 milligrams of sodium per liter after softening), which he characterizes as "extreme." Dr. Schroeder points out that anyone who drinks that water would disrupt a diet aimed at restricting sodium intake to 200 milligrams or even 500 milligrams of sodium per day. Some waters, of course, add only a few milligrams of sodium a day.

"If one suspects that tap water contains enough sodium to affect the total intake," says Dr. Schroeder, "analysis and decision on using bottled water for drinking and cooking should be made. Values for sodium in municipal water can be obtained from treatment plants." Now this presupposes two rather unlikely possibilities: (a) that the average householder would get to wondering about the sodium value of his tap water, when he is probably unaware that it is being softened by the city, hence unaware that excess sodium is coming his way; (b) that he would take the time to call the treatment plant for the information, or have the background needed to relate the information they give him to its importance in *his* life.

Most Americans are not likely to suspect danger from softened water. Rather they would be inclined to give the water bureau a rousing vote of thanks if it were to soften the municipal water supply.

In the *Journal of the American Medical Association*

(December 12, 1959) the two most common methods of water softening are discussed: the soda-lime method and the ion-exchange (zeolite) type. With the soda-lime process, which is most used by large cities who soften the entire municipal water supply, the water is substantially free of sodium. However, smaller communities and private homes usually use the ion-echange method, and the resultant water has a "substantial sodium" in it as a result of the softening process. The *American Journal of Public Health* (October, 1955) printed the conclusion that water softened by the ion-exchange method might contain more sodium than is desirable for some high blood pressure patients.

In the early 1950's the city of Toledo, Ohio, carried on experiments to discover the best way to soften the city's water supply. After spending $770,000 on the project, it was dropped. Reason: the local industries complained that their heating equipment was being ruined by unabsorbed chemicals from the softening process. Not a word about what these same chemicals could be doing to the people of Toledo; it was the industrial equipment which must be protected!

A further warning about the use of water softeners comes to us from a book called *Trace Elements in Foods* by G. W. Monier-Williams, O.B.E., M.A., Ph.D., F.R.I.C., formerly of the Ministry of Health in England (John Wiley & Sons Inc., New York, 1949). Discussing the use of aluminum cooking utensils, Dr. Monier-Williams says: "Aluminum is not attacked by distilled water, whether hot or cold, but hard water corrodes it slightly and may become cloudy with suspended aluminum hydroxide. London tap water boiled in aluminum saucepans and allowed to stand overnight takes up from 8 to 20 parts per million of the metal. Water softened by base exchange processes, using zeolite regenerated with salt, may be extremely corrosive to aluminum, and kettles in which such water is used have a comparatively short life."

Of course such a situation is bad news for human health. Yet, how many people drinking softened water have a doctor who will consider the type of water they are drinking in relation to their worsening illness? How many people have become ill due to increased sodium in their tissues, and have no inkling that the softened water they drink to help them take their pills is the very reason for their problem?

Minerals

It is clear that soft water, while more pleasant to use, is short on many minerals. It is reasonable to suspect that one or a combination of these minerals are valuable to continued good circulation in the body. When one uses water that has a shortage of them, and if one should eat a diet in which they are not adequately supplied, it is not surprising that the shortage should make itself felt in some physical breakdown.

Water with as many natural minerals as possible is the best for drinking. If one should discover that one's local water supply is very soft, one should make every effort to eat mineral-rich foods and to include a mineral food supplement in the diet to make up for any possible loss.

Recently, science has been establishing that mineral nutrition—in some cases involving quantities so slight you need a microscope to see them at all—is fundamental to heart health. Tiny traces of such minerals as chromium and cadmium, selenium and zinc, are believed by many researchers to often make the difference between healthy and sick hearts. Longer and better known are the relationship of calcium to a regular heartbeat, magnesium and phosphorus to proper absorption and use of calcium, and potassium to maintain the slight alkalinity a healthy heart requires.

This makes a wide array of minerals your heart needs. To prevent blood pressure and circulatory disorders, you should know a bit about the most important minerals and how to get them through a natural diet and appropriate supplements.

The relatively new approach to heart problems—preventive cardiology—spotlights two common minerals, potassium and magnesium, as especially valuable for preserving the health of the heart muscle. According to Eors Bajusz, M.D., Ph.D., of Bio-Research Institute in Cambridge, Massachusetts, this area is the most common place of injury in cardiac diseases. The nutrition present there might explain why one individual has the ability to resist heart disease while another develops fatal degenerative changes in the heart muscle when he is exposed to the same stresses. The article in the *Medical Tribune* (February 29, 1968) states that apparently variations in such dietary elements as glucose, lactate, pyruvate, fatty acids and amino acids do not play a major role in determining which heart will suffer and which will not. Yet, says Bajusz, "Certain electrolytes, especially potassium and magnesium, seem to be key factors in this respect." He reported:

"When fed with experimental diets deficient in one or both of these minerals, laboratory animals suffered severe disturbances in cardiac function, degeneration of myocardial fibers and cardiac death. Even today, scant attention is paid to the large number of experimental studies indicating that even a transient decrease in myocardial potassium and magnesium concentrations is of considerable importance because it generally sensitizes the heart muscle to cardio-toxic influences and, conversely, a dietary excess of K (potassium) and/or Mg (magnesium) protects the heart against the induction of morphologic abnormalities. . . ." The doctor was able to demonstrate that giving these two mineral salts to laboratory animals prevented the development of 18 types of potentially fatal heart problems.

The article concludes, significantly, that a large percentage of patients admitted to hospitals reveal some degree of potassium deficiency and that in general the average potassium intake of Americans is much lower than they think it is. "Under potentially cardio-toxic influences, the nutritional requirements of cardiac muscle cells increase as far as the need of K or Mg ions is concerned, and the customary dietary intake is insufficient to satisfy this increased demand." It is suggested that the two minerals act together to protect the heart.

Potassium

Potassium is an essential mineral that is easy to forget, and whose lack may be one reason the death rate from heart disease keeps climbing so steadily in the United States. The L. Peter Cogan Foundation, of New York, issued a report in November, 1959, suggesting that national heart disease rates are inversely tied to the amount of potassium in a nation's traditional foods. Where potassium-rich foods are frequently consumed (Japan, Scandinavia, Italy, France, Germany, Netherlands and Switzerland) the heart disease rates are low, compared with countries whose diets are not particularly rich in potassium (United States, Australia, Canada, New Zealand, United Kingdom). The Japanese eat plenty of potassium in seafood and seaweed (kelp), and the potassium-rich mushrooms that appear frequently in their national dishes. Italians are fond of seafood; olive oil and grape wine (both good potassium sources) are part of every meal.

In the *New York State Journal of Medicine* (July 15, 1957) J. Yerushalmy, Ph.D., and Herman Hilleboe, M.D., presented evidence from 22 countries showing that the presumed association between the percentage of fat calories available for consumption in the national diet and mortality from arteriosclerosis and other heart ailments is not valid. "It is true that the Japanese and Italian diets contain a much smaller percentage of animal fats than the United States. On the other hand, the diets of Swedes, Danes and Norwegians contain approximately the same proportion of animal fat as that of the Americans, but the mortality rate in these countries is just a little over a third of that in America." The Cogan Foundation report suggests that the potassium rich diet of seafoods and mushrooms consumed in the Scandinavian countries may be a mitigating factor.

The report reinforces its point by showing that potassium deficiency can have a heavy influence on the ordinary workings of the heart. Dr. Samuel Bellet, of the University of Pennsylvania, in his book *Potassium: Cardiac Aspects, The Role of Potassium in Health and Disease* (1952) writes, "Animals fed diets low in potassium failed to grow at a normal rate. After several weeks the heart shows evidence of myocardial necrosis. . . . A heart lesion may be produced in four days by a diet low in potassium and high in sodium chloride, together with injections of desoxycorticosteroneacetate." A famous heart researcher, Dr. Hans Selye of the

University of Montreal, performed experiments on rats, injecting them with potassium and magnesium to protect them against sudden extreme stress. Those not treated in this way developed damage in the heart muscle and died.

Investigators are still working to find out exactly what it could be in the potassium-rich foods that has such a beneficial influence against heart disease. One important consideration is potassium's effect on the skeletal muscles which contain about six times as much potassium as sodium. It influences the contractibility of the smooth, skeletal and cardiac muscle and profoundly affects the nerve tissues. It could be that potassium's greatest contribution to heart health is its maintenance of the heart's muscle power.

There is also strong evidence that potassium serves as an anti-toxic agent in the protection of the heart. Dr. P. Prioreschi, writing in the *Canadian Medical Association Journal* (April 29, 1967), stated that while it has been established that a number of substances widely found in our environment are actively toxic to the heart, one particular mineral nutrient—potassium—was able in almost every case to counteract the effects of these poisons and prevent heart attacks.

Potassium was called a treatment for exhaustion and fatigue by Dr. P. E. Formica in *Current Therapeutic Research* (March, 1962). He administered potassium and magnesium salts of aspartic acid to 84 housewives and 16 men who had complained of headache, insomnia, back pain, marital difficulties and boredom for weeks, some for years. At the end of the trial, 87 percent of the subjects had responded favorably. Among other results, marital difficulties decreased. Sexual responsiveness, often diminished in middle-aged people due partly to fatigue, improved in these patients. Dr. Formica concluded that "Potassium and magnesium salts of aspartic acid, although not a panacea, afford the first fully, first truly effective physiological treatment for chronic fatigue whether or not it is associated with organic disease."

Major deficiencies of potassium, so serious that they are obvious upon examination, are rare. But it doesn't take a major deficiency to cause trouble. Even minor shortages of potassium can bring on vague weakness, impairment of neuromuscular function, poor reflexes and mental confusion. The muscles become soft and saggy and healthy cell growth is sluggish, when optimum potassium is missing. Dry skin in mature persons and acne in adolescents are also warning signals that more potassium is needed.

And keep in mind the effect of a hot climate on the body's potassium supply. As Dr. James L. Schamadan and W. D. Snively pointed out in *Industrial Medicine and Surgery* (December 1967), high heat causes excessive losses of potassium, since potassium is one of the major ingredients of perspiration. Potassium is so intimately involved with normal heart action, the authors remind us, that two Los Angeles physicians—Drs. Sidney Franklin and Daniel Simmons of the UCLA Medical School—have suggested that heart trouble can be predicted from a change in the normal potassium levels.

A striking correlation between potassium deficit and heat exhaustion was noted during a prolonged heat wave which involved the Central Great Plains and Mississippi Valley areas in July, 1966. Temperatures never went under 90 degrees Fahrenheit for three weeks and hovered above 100 degrees for more than a week. Coincidental power shortages prevented adequate air conditioning. During this time more than 150 deaths were officially attributed to "heat prostration" or "heat exhaustion." An examination of hospital records showed that many of the victims had depressed serum potassium levels.

In every case, perspiration had been excessive in the days before collapse. Many who had cardiovascular disease, were taking thiazide or digitalis or both. Thiazide is known to encourage potassium losses, and coupled with excessive perspiration and a lowered potassium intake due to lack of appetite in the heat, set the stage for severe potassium deficits. Observers believe that this potassium deficit could have contributed heavily to the heat-stress disease that killed these people.

Schamadan and Snively report on other workers' findings of heart failure cases and increased incidence of heart trouble in your people in high-temperature areas who had no previous history of heart disease. The researchers feel that potassium depletion may have been the reason for heart trouble here too. When Schamadan studied heat-tolerance problems in Vietnam he noticed that two pilots showed exceptional ability to maintain high levels of performance over long periods, in spite of the heat. Both of the men consumed large amounts of ketchup with almost every meal. Plain tomato ketchup contains quite large amounts of potassium.

At the 48th Annual Session of the American College of Physicians in San Francisco (April, 1967), Drs. R. M. Vertel and J. P. Knochel pointed out the possible relationship between potassium depletion and high incidence of heat stroke among otherwise healthy soldiers in basic training and football players in pre-season conditioning. They warned strongly against the indiscriminate use of salt tablets, which can promote the exchange of sodium for potassium. In the hot countries of Indonesia and Nigeria, they point out, peasants—who have a daily diet high in potassium but quite low in sodium—resist heat injuries characterized by electrolyte disturbances, fever, etc.

Persons whose work exposes them to high heat for extended periods are clearly among those who should pay special attention to their potassium intake. So are the country's sunbathers! Above all, men and women who have experienced any cardiac difficulties should make sure of a plentiful supply of potassium in their diets.

There would be no problem in this country in our getting enough potassium if our diet habits were pegged more to fresh, natural foods than the processed ones we favor. There is plenty of potassium in meats, seeds, green leafy vegetables and fruits. But the popular choices are the highly processed items. Raw peaches contain 880 milligrams of potassium per 100 grams. Can them and the reading goes down to 450. Frozen peaches contain only 133 milligrams of potassium per hundred grams. Wheat germ contains 780 milligrams of potassium per 100 grams, while self-rising, enriched, fortified, all-purpose wheat flour has 90. The popular fig bar cookies contain absolutely no potassium, but dried figs have a reading of 780 milligrams per 100 grams.

Dr. W. A. Krehl, writing in *Nutrition in Clinical Medicine* (August 22, 1966) said, "If food habits had always been sound, the event of potassium deficiency and depletion would not have developed as a major medical problem." He affirms that poor dietary habits, restricted diet selection, misuse and inappropriate choice of foods are all to blame for any potassium deficiences that exist.

You can go after a better potassium balance in your system by following a few simple rules. Try to be sure there is a good amount of meat in your diet every day and don't overshadow it by useless carbohydrate foods. You'll find squash and organ meats are valuable. Use salads at every opportunity along with any other fresh fruit or vegetable in season. Cut your salt intake. The sodium in salt is constantly at war with potassium for the control of the cells. When sodium takes over, a poisonous condition exists that leads to death of the cells and the eventual destruction of tissues. Supplements that can provide extra potassium are bone meal, brewer's yeast, sunflower seeds, desiccated liver and wheat germ.

If maintaining a good potassium supply is indeed the key to a healthy heart, it is a goal that's easy enough to accomplish. Review your daily eating habits and take the steps necessary to improve your personal odds against getting heart trouble.

Calcium and Magnesium

That the human heart is an unbelievably efficient type of pump, able to push incredible quantities of fluid and to work continuously, day and night, without ever resting, is a phenomenon that has long been recognized. Not so long known and far from universally recognized is the fact that the mineral nutrient calcium is indispensable to the ability of the heart to keep working. Failure to recognize this might be compared to understanding that a gasoline explosion turns the drive shaft of a car but not knowing that the gasoline will not explode unless it has a spark plug to ignite it.

Dr. Winifred Nayler of the Baker Medical Research Institute describes the process in *Heart Journal* (March, 1967) as an electrochemical process that takes place within each cell of the heart. On the outer surface of each heart tissue cell there is a thin filament known as actin. The actin reaches with a kind of magnetic attraction toward the center of the cell, shortening its length. The result of many cells shortening at one time is contraction of the muscle. And it is calcium, fed to the actin by the bloodstream, that provides both the stimulus and the means by which the actin does its work. A shortage of calcium must inevitably result in a weakened heartbeat, which can be sped up by drug stimulants but cannot be strengthened, as long as the calcium is deficient. Even this simple explanation, we believe, points out the folly of treating a weak heartbeat with drugs, at least until the ability to absorb calcium and the quantity of calcium in the diet has been checked and corrected.

To continue our analogy, however, when you understand that it takes a spark plug to ignite your gasoline, that isn't the end of the story. It also takes ignition points to direct electrical energy to the right spark plug at the right time. And, as Dr. Nayler tells us, while calcium is fundamentally necessary to the heartbeat, the calcium will not do what it is supposed to do unless it is controlled in its turn by a sufficient quantity of magnesium in the system.

The reason for this, Dr. Nayler says, is that it is necessary for the actin alternately to absorb and release calcium. If it could not do both, the heart would either contract and stay contracted or else refuse to contract at all. To create a system in which the heart can keep contracting and relaxing alternately requires that it be a very busy living chemical laboratory. And it is magnesium that seems to be the key element that actually regulates the heartbeat. How does it do it? By providing a tiny positive electrical charge that repels calcium, pushing it to the opposite side of the individual cell and reversing the contraction that has just taken place. Throughout the body, magnesium seems to be the mineral of basic importance in this matter of controlling the manner in which electrical charges are utilized to induce the passage of materials in and out of cells.

Nor is the heart the only portion of the circulatory system that is affected and, in effect, controlled by whether we obtain enough magnesium in our diets.

Throughout our system, all muscular tissues are designed to be able both to contract and to relax, and if either function fails there is trouble. Hypertension, or high blood pressure, is characterized by an excessive contraction or inability to relax the muscles surrounding the walls of arteries. It was reported in the *Journal of the American Medical Association* (February 22, 1965) by Dr. R. H. Seller that magnesium salts induced these muscles to relax and had therefore been found effective as a treatment for high blood pressure.

Similarly, in experimenting on the cellular metabolism with possible treatments for arteriosclerosis, Dr. T. Shimamoto reported in the *American Heart Journal* in 1959 that he was able to reduce swelling and consequent constriction of arterial walls with magnesium salts. According to Dr. Mildred Seelig (*American Journal of Clinical Nutrition,* June, 1964) there is a direct relationship between the amount of magnesium in the diet and ability to avoid high blood pressure. Dr. Seelig regards the difference in magnesium consumption as an important reason why there are far fewer heart attacks among orientals than there are in the west.

The study of magnesium and its many roles in human metabolism is only in its infancy. Until very recent years, this was the forgotten mineral. It was known to be essential, but nobody had any idea what it really does within the system nor did anyone seem to care much.

Today it is a different matter. As the science of biochemistry continues to develop, scientists have come to realize how important is the long-known fact that our bodies are constantly generating tiny electrical impulses and discharging them. Every movement, external or internal, is triggered by such impulses transmitted along nerves. Without our electrical systems, there could be no life whatsoever. And so, today, we are compelled to recognize that if magnesium is the primary regulator of the electrical activity within our bodies, then magnesium is obviously of far greater importance to health and life itself than anybody had guessed even ten years ago.

Dr. Mildred Seelig, previously cited, calculated that the average American falls short by 200 milligrams a day or more of the optimal amount of magnesium one should consume for good health. Present in many foods, magnesium in unfortunately extremely sensitive to heat and easily lost during the processing of foods. People who eat raw and unprocessed foods probably get enough. How many in America do? How many in America even find it possible?

Therein, perhaps, lies the answer to the riddle of why so many Americans get heart attacks, high blood pressure, and strokes and why these diseases are on the increase in western Europe. Nor is the circulatory system the only group of organs to which you will be giving a health boost if you are careful to add more magnesium to your diet. Even among essential nutrients, this one seems just a bit more essential.

Chromium Good, Cadmium Bad

Without realizing it man has subjected himself to an experiment in trace element imbalance over the past 500 to 1,000 years, and the result of that experiment could be certain degenerative disease, Henry. A. Schroeder, M.D., whom we have previously quoted, told participants at the 1968 American Heart Association meeting. By mining metals from the earth man has disturbed the world-wide distribution of trace elements in air, water and food, Dr. Schroeder noted. Civilized man has received the most exposure to that trace element imbalance, the research said, because of air and water pollution, food processing and other factors.

In order to try to determine the exact result of man's trace element experiment upon himself, Dr. Schroeder and his associates built a small animal laboratory on top of a mountain, where it could be kept free from pollution. No metals were used in its construction. In its maintenance, air and water are carefully filtered, and no visitors—who may be carrying contaminants on their clothes—are permitted. Animals raised in the laboratory are given diets free of some elements under study. Carefully controlled amounts of the desired elements are added to the animals' diet as desired. Dr. Schroeder also reported on the trace element analysis of 180,000 different samples of human tissue, collected from both primitive and civilized people from all over the world. The purpose of the human sampling was to study the relative trace element content of various organs and body tissues of civilized as compared to primitive peoples.

The two elements which Dr. Schroeder has focused the most attention on are cadmium and chromium. His work has shown that cadmium may be the cause of the puzzling "essential" high blood pressure that troubles about five percent of adult Americans and is one of the serious diseases of aging. Neither animals nor human beings have cadmium in their tissues at birth, Dr. Schroeder reports. Rats kept free of cadmium at the mountaintop laboratory didn't develop hypertension as they grew older, but the condition did appear in rats who were fed small amounts of that trace element. When the cadmium-fed hypertensive rats were fed a chemical capable of removing the cadmium from their systems, their blood pressure declined to normal ranges. Dr. Schroeder has found that cadmium builds up in human tissue as people grow older, but he has yet to provide the conclusive evidence that cadmium is the cause of essential hypertension in human beings. "It will take 100 people working in this field to provide all the answers," he commented.

Chromium, on the other hand, could be described as a "good" element, it was reported for the first time. Americans are born with high tissue levels of chromium, but the amount declines as they get older. Hardening of the arteries and diabetes are less severe in areas of the world where body chromium remains high—places where people live a more primitive life. Laboratory rats kept deficient in chromium had sharply higher incidence of atherosclerosis and diabetes. Rats given chromium for their lifetimes lived significantly longer than others and were almost completely free of signs of atherosclerosis.

Differences in the eating habits of civilized and primitive people were suggested as the cause of the variations in trace element balance, and possibly are the cause of cardiovascular diseases. Refining of grain is known to concentrate cadmium—the harmful element—while the same process reduces chromium values. Refining of sugar removes chromium. Dr. Schroeder also presented evidence that the more sugar a person consumes, the greater is the body's metabolic demand for chromium. Since refined sugar doesn't contain the element, depletion results. Coffee and tea—common beverages in civilized countries—are known to be high in harmful cadmium. The super-heating of food during processing was also suggested as a possible cause of chromium loss.

Vanadium Protects the Heart

Scientists aren't sure whether vanadium, a trace mineral, keeps excessive cholesterol from forming, or breaks it down when it has formed; perhaps it does both. The question came to the fore when researchers discovered vanadium abundant in the hard drinking waters of certain areas of the southwest, the very areas where death rates from degenerative heart disease are lowest in the United States. It is barely present in the soft water of the Coastal and Great Lakes States, the states, as the researchers suspected, where death rates from heart disease are highest. In a speech to the American Association for the Advancement of Science (December 29, 1961) Dr. William H. Strain suggested that "There are very significant geographical variations in death rates for all causes and for cardiovascular diseases that may be due to variable intake of trace elements, especially vanadium and zinc."

A great deal has been written about the possibility that all life originated in the oceans, billions of years ago. If this is true, the role of sea minerals in the physiology of man deserves more attention. In his book, *Sea Within* (Lippincott), W. D. Snively makes the point that the extracellular fluid (about 30 percent of the human body) is essentially diluted sea water. Of course the body has its own mechanisms for keeping the composition of this inner ocean constant, but deficiencies of various sorts can develop when there are dietary shortages of specific minerals.

A 1956 study of the Scandinavian countries showed that the death rate from heart disease among these countries is exceptionally low. Scientists researched all types of data about these rich diet nations, trying to find an explanation for this happy state. Consideration of the consumption of fat, meat and milk in each country showed no relationship of these food factors to the death rate. The doctors found that one environmental influence that might vary is the intake of trace elements.

In sea-side Scandinavian countries, ocean fish are eaten in large quantities and sea salt (rich in a variety of trace elements) is used for preserving fish, for cattle and for household consumption. To add credibility to the importance of the water-surrounded situation of these countries, Professor

Niels Dungal reported in 1953 on 2,200 autopsies in Iceland. The arteries of the Icelanders, at age 60, compared well with the arteries of Austrians at age 40. William H. Strain, Ph.D., suggests that their lack of cholesterol accumulation might be credited to the ingestion of vanadium and other trace minerals.

Lack of trace elements in the soil is common to certain parts of this country. As we have seen, the drinking water varies from very hard to very soft, and then the mineral constituents of hard water vary from place to place as well. Milk, frequently mentioned as a source of trace minerals, reflects both the soil and water that make up the environment of the cow, and its mineral composition is extremely variable. Vanadium is not present in meat in measurable amounts, but it is found in varying quantities in vegetables.

Marine life is the most reliable source of vanadium, in Dr. Strain's opinion. Particularly good sources are herring and sardines. Larger fish show variations in the content of vanadium. However, it seems reasonable that "all ocean fish contain some vanadium, but . . . the amount varies with the species."

Circulatory disturbances are frequently caused by a pile-up of cholesterol in the blood vessels. But cholesterol is a valuable constituent of the brain, spinal cord and other portions of the nervous system; so the need is to regulate cholesterol formation rather than to inhibit it completely. Presumably when the body has the proper equipment, it manages this regulation very nicely. Vanadium is part of this natural regulating system. Researchers have demonstrated that the presence of vanadium in the brain inhibits cholesterol formation. They have also shown that the formation of cholesterol in the human central nervous system can be cut by administering vanadium orally.

J. T. Mountain and associates reporting in *Federation Proceedings* (18, 425, 1959) described an elaborate study with rabbits that showed vanadium added to the standard diet at premeasured levels lowered free cholesterol and fat content of the liver in the rabbits. When vanadium was added to a one percent cholesterol diet, it held down the elevation of free and total cholesterols in the plasma; when rabbits were fed cholesterol to raise the plasma level, and then the cholesterol was omitted from the diet, the presence of vanadium in the diet was given credit for a faster return to normal cholesterol readings than occurred when no vanadium was furnished. Mountain and his associates concluded that vanadium both inhibits the formation of cholesterol and speeds the destruction of it.

The use of vanadium in humans for limiting the cholesterol count has been considered both as a preventive and as a type of therapy. G. L. Curran and R. L. Costello reported in the *Journal of Experimental Medicine* (103, 49, 1956) that six weeks of administering vanadium resulted in statistically significant lowering of the serum total and free cholesterol levels. The vanadium lowered tissue cholesterol stores in four out of five men studied. A small group of vanadium workers were observed, and, compared with a control group, the workers had a significantly lower cholesterol value.

It is interesting that scientists found it difficult to decide on a simple, reliable method of measuring vanadium levels in man. Although 90 percent of ingested vanadium is eliminated in the urine, determining the urinary levels of vanadium in large communities is impracticable. A simpler method recently presented itself. Changes in the levels of vanadium show up in the hair. Dr. Strain suggests that, with this simple means of measurement, a more elaborate program for studying the important relationship between vanadium intake and cardiovascular death could be undertaken.

Dr. Strain points out that an overdose of vanadium, even in a synthetic form, is difficult to get. However, all nutritional elements, including vanadium, are best taken in the form that nature provides. Fish, of course, is an excellent source. Unfortunately, few Americans make fish any part of the diet and if they do it is too occasional to be dependable. As we have seen, milk and vegetables are also unreliable sources of vanadium, because the content of this mineral varies from one location to the next, one cow or plant to the next. It is revealing to see, then, that seaweed is frequently on the menu in the Scandinavian countries, the same ones that have such a good record for controlling heart disease. Seaweed, preferably kelp, is an ideal source of vanadium and other important trace minerals.

The brown seaweeds are the commonest, and the ones used most widely for food. Just like other plants, they contain carbohydrates, protein and other nutrients. There is some vitamin A and some of the B vitamins, but the vitamin C content of seaweed is comparable to that of many vegetables and fruits. For many Eskimos, seaweed was once the chief source of vitamin C. One test showed a vitamin C content of 5 to 140 milligrams per 100 grams of wet seaweed. Oranges contain about 50 milligrams per 100 grams.

But the main attraction of seaweed is its mineral content. Plants that grow on land take up minerals from the soil. The same is true of sea plants, and the sea is the richest source of all minerals. W. A. P. Black, writing in the *Proceedings of Nutrition Society of England* (12, 32, 1953), tells us that the ash of seaweed may be from 10 to as high as 50 percent. This means that if you burn seaweed, you may have half the volume of the seaweed left as minerals. Compare this to some other foods: carrots leave an ash of 1 percent; apples have a mineral ash of .3 percent; almonds, 3.0 percent. Black writes, "It can be said that seaweed contains all the elements that have so far been shown to play an important part in the physiological processes of man. In a balanced diet, therefore, they would appear to be an excellent mineral supplement."

Don't leave your mineral nutrition to chance. Scientists have proven that you need vanadium. Make sure you get it by eating all the fish you can, or, to play safe, put some kelp in your daily diet.

Copper Strengthens the Blood Vessels

Copper is one of those trace minerals that is key to life—you would die without it—yet it can be poisonous if injected even in small amounts beyond those required by your body. Usually your body maintains a nice balance, so you should never go on a crash program to either eliminate or increase your copper intake.

Of the many essential functions of copper in the body's metabolism, we will talk here of its role in the prevention of heart disease. Recent research has revealed the importance of this trace mineral to the tensile strength of the coronary blood vessels.

Dr. William H. Carnes, Professor of Pathology at the University of Utah College of Medicine, has observed a cardiovascular syndrome in animals, caused by insufficient dietary intake of copper. His discovery, reported in the *Medical Tribune* (August 15, 1968), sheds new light on the importance of copper in the normal development of vascular connective tissue. Dr. Carnes described the syndrome at the 1968 Conference on Trace Substances as one marked by internal hemorrhage due to rupture of the aorta (the large artery leading from the heart) and coronary vessels. He traced the disease to a defect in synthesis of vascular elastin apparently brought about by a deficiency in a copper-containing enzyme.

In the experiments described by Dr. Carnes, pigs were weaned at two to five days of life and put on a diet of dilute canned evaporated milk which is low in copper content. These animals soon developed characteristic cardiovascular lesions, most commonly of the aorta and coronary arteries. Death from cardiovascular rupture or from heart failure occurred usually between three and four months of age. However, lesions could be corrected and death prevented simply by supplementing the diet with copper after a deficiency had appeared.

After studying the mechanical properties of the aorta in the affected animals, Dr. Carnes concluded that rupture was due to reduced tensile strength or reduced extensibility of the vessel. In other words, the coronary vessel, instead of easily stretching to accommodate its load, would break like a balloon that is stretched beyond its ability to expand.

Dr. Carnes noted that while an extreme copper deficiency like that induced in the animals would be unlikely in humans, under some circumstances there might be a metabolic block in copper enzyme synthesis or a missing co-factor—for example a lack of pyridoxine (B_6) in a copper pyridoxal enzyme.

Dr. Boyd O'Dell of the University of Missouri,

Department of Agricultural Chemistry, another conference participant, found similarities between the lesions occurring in copper-deficient animals and those seen in human subjects. As a result of O'Dell's findings, Dr. John H. Henzel, also of the University of Missouri, performed copper assays on specimens obtained from patients requiring resection of diseased abdominal aortas because of occlusive or aneurysmal disease. Nine patients were studied.

In those patients with aortic aneurysm, the copper content was significantly less. For instance, the average copper concentration in specimens from patients with atherosclerosis but no aneurysm was 26.3 ppm. (parts per million). For patients with both atherosclerosis and aneurysms, it was 21.2 ppm. whereas for those with aortic aneurysms without visible evidence of atherosclerosis, copper content was only 14.2 ppm. This would lead us to suspect that in those patients whose hearts were dangerously threatened yet who had no evidence of atherosclerosis, the usual precursor to heart disease, that the lack of copper in the tissue, by causing a decrease in the elasticity of the blood vessel, was a prime cause of the aneurysm.

Earl Frieden in a scholarly report "The Biochemistry of Copper" (*Scientific American,* May, 1968) reports that "A copper deficiency can result in the weakening of the walls of certain blood vessels, notably the aorta, rendering the vessels susceptible to aneurysms and rupture."

The trace mineral zinc apparently plays a role in adjusting the amount of copper used in body metabolism, according to an April 1968 report by Dr. Darrell R. Van Campen, of the United States Department of Agriculture. Fortunately, both zinc and copper occur in a healthy balance in foods easily included in the diet, such as seafoods and organ meats.

Zinc

"Recognition of zinc deficiency as a problem in man has taken a long time," a pioneer in zinc research, Walter J. Pories, M.D., told a gathering of the prestigious American Association for the Advancement of Science in December 1968.

The speaker, a professor at the School of Medicine and Dentistry of the University of Rochester, went on to say:

"Within the past few years, investigators have demonstrated in rapid succession that zinc deficiency is common in man, and that this deficiency is a critical factor in impaired growth, delayed healing, and chronic disease."

Of the chronic diseases related to zinc deficiencies, Dr. Pories singled out atherosclerosis as "the most common cause of death in the United States . . . one of the most vexing chronic diseases in medical research since it seems partly an environmental and preventable disease."

Now it is true, as Dr. Pories said, that among

scientists engaged in research on zinc and other trace metals, zinc deficiency in our population is recognized as a serious environmental problem. But how widely recognized is this fact by the people who determine the content of our food and water? How many physicians are likely to consider zinc deficiency in the treatment of their patients with heart disease?

The first clue relating zinc deficiency to atherosclerosis came to Dr. Pories and his colleagues during a trace metal survey of patients with different diseases in the University of Rochester Medical Center. "Persons with atherosclerosis uniformly demonstrated low zinc values."

Other investigators have come up with similar findings—for example, Dr. Bert L. Vallee, of Harvard Medical School, and scientists at the Minsk Medical Institute of Russia. All confirm that people with hardening of the arteries almost always are zinc deficient.

At the 1967 convention of the American Medical Association, Dr. Pories reported on the use of zinc therapy in the treatment of patients suffering from serious vascular disorders. Twelve patients with advanced or inoperable vascular disease were treated, some for more than two years, with oral supplements of 220 mg. zinc sulfate, three times daily. "Though the series is small," said Dr. Pories, "we are delighted with our findings. All patients have shown considerable improvement and none has had any further vascular catastrophes or progression of atherosclerosis. More important than this nice improvement in these inoperable patients with advanced atherosclerosis, is the thesis that this illness is an environmental disease partly due to an *easily correctable* deficiency."

How the zinc operates to help the patient Dr. Pories explained as follows "A tiny amount of zinc is present in enzymes essential to the original growth of mammalian organisms and also, it seems, to the regrowth of destroyed or damaged tissues. The effectiveness of zinc therapy in the treatment of this arterial disease is probably related to healing. Pathologists have found that the degenerative changes in the blood vessels are initiated by injury or by accumulation of fatty deposits which foster breakdown and ulceration of the tissues of the blood vessels."

The healing power of zinc came to light quite by accident during studies in which wounded laboratory rats eating food contaminated with compounds of zinc, healed faster than others not getting the compound. Prompted by this revelation, Dr. Pories and his colleague, Dr. Strain (whom we have quoted earlier on the value of trace metals), tested the effectiveness of zinc on surgical patients at Wright-Patterson Air Force Base in Ohio. They gave daily capsules of zinc sulfate to ten young airmen who were undergoing a type of surgery that is always slow to heal. The rate of healing proved three times better in patients getting zinc. No toxic effects were observed in tests ranging from 43 to 61 days.

The effective role played by zinc in the healing of arterial lesions, when considered in the light of the geography of atherosclerosis, lends considerable weight to the suggestion that mineral imbalance may well be a strong causative factor and that this disease is not necessarily the inevitable concomitant of growing old. "Although vascular disease is a frequent finding in an older person," says W. C. Manion ("Aging Circulation," *Mil. Med.,* July, 1963), "it should not be assumed that vascular disease is a natural and normal sequence of aging."

If atherosclerosis were merely a degenerative disease and not related to environment, it should be evenly distributed across the United States in proportion to the aging population. This is not the case. Furthermore, age and youth—in themselves—do not determine the onslaught of the disease. Centenarians have been reported where careful examination has shown little or no vascular disease, while other patients have presented with severe sclerotic lesions in the first few months or years of life (H. Hirsch, cited by Korenshevsky, *Physiological and Pathological Ageing,* Basel, Switzerland, 1961).

The environmental factor is further borne out by the fact that in some countries atherosclerosis is a rarity while in the United States it has reached epidemic proportions, eventually killing three out of every four males. Even within the United States, there are large geographic differences in the death rates from cardiovascular disease. In the surveys of the U. S. Public Health Service, it has become apparent that the highest death rates are near the two sea coasts, the Gulf of Mexico, the Great Lakes, and along the Mississippi Basin. It appears that the high death rates are associated with areas of high water drainage, where the minerals have been leached from the soils or where compounds, washing down with the rivers, could be binding minerals into a biologically unavailable form, Dr. Pories said.

In an attempt to explain the regional variations, investigators in Japan, Great Britain and the United States have pointed out that areas with soft water have significantly higher cardiovascular death rates than areas where the drinking water contains more mineral matter.

Minerals are also leached from the soils in the presence of artificial fertilizers and poisonous sprays, says Dr. Andre Voisin in his book *Soil, Grass, and Cancer* (C. Lockwood, Great Britain, 1959).

In fact, the Trace Element Committee of the Council on Fertilizer Application has identified 32 of the 50 states as zinc deficient. Many of these have been shown to be the high mortality states in a United States Public Health Service Survey.

The zinc deficiency of the soil is carried over to our food plants, and to the cattle which man depends upon for the staff of life. Add to this soil and water deficiency the fact that, like every other mineral element, zinc is concentrated in the bran and germ portions of cereal grains—the parts that are removed in the refining process and not replaced in the so-called enriching program—and you have some understanding of why atherosclerosis is becoming a national tragedy.

But the exciting and encouraging note sounded

High Zinc Foods

Food	*Parts per Million of Zinc*
Barley	27
Beef	20-50
Beets	28
Cabbage	2-15
Carrots	5-36
Clams	20
Corn	25
Eggs, dry, whole	55
Egg yolk	26-40
Herring	700-1200
Liver, beef	30-85
Milk, cow	4-30
Oatmeal	140
Oysters	1600
Pumpkin seeds	38
Peanut butter	20
Peas	30-50
Rice	15
Spinach	3-9
Sunflower seeds	66
Syrup, maple	52-105
Wheat bran	140
Yeast, brewer's	80

by Dr. Pories—that atherosclerosis may well be due to an "easily correctable deficiency" is one which brings to those who are careful of their nutrition, great hope for a healthier tomorrow.

Indeed, the developing knowledge of trace minerals and their role in metabolism may well provide the solution to the heart disease problem.

CHAPTER X

Vitamins and the Circulatory System

ALTHOUGH it has long been known that the lack of certain organic chemical substances called vitamins can cause such diseases as rickets, scurvy beriberi, pellagra, etc., only recently has attention been given to the role of vitamins in the health of the circulatory system. As might be expected, controversy is compounded in the fields of chemistry, nutrition, biology, physiology, metabolism, and offshoots of these. The result is that specialists who accept the fact that vitamin D can cure rickets deny that vitamin E is useful in treating heart disease or circulatory disorders.

Yet ample evidence has been accumulated on the role of various vitamins in the circulatory system, and thoughtful people can draw their own conclusions.

The Vitamin B Complex

There are many parts of the vitamin B complex that have been shown by medical research to be of value in the prevention and cure of atherosclerosis. Choline is one of them. Choline is a lipotropic agent, which means that it combines readily with fats or oils, and thus hastens the removal of fat deposits. We have seen in previous chapters the dangerous effect of fatty deposits on the walls of the arteries. In the *Proceedings of the Society of Biology and Medicine* (73: 37-38, 1950) there is an article describing a study of the effect of choline on 230 patients, done by Drs. L. M. Morrison, and W. F. Gonzales of the College of Medical Evangelists, Los Angeles, California. It was summarized in *Modern Medicine* as follows: "Half the patients were given conventional medication but no choline after discharge from the hospital; the other half received choline daily for one to three years. Among the untreated patients, the three-year death toll was about 30 percent, while only 12 percent of the choline-treated patients died."

These patients were given synthetically made choline. If, however, you take brewer's yeast or desiccated liver you would be getting choline in its natural form, which is much safer. In this experiment the aim was to give a maximum dose of 32 grams of choline daily by mouth, but many patients suffered side reactions such as gastroenteritis, dizzy spells and unpleasant body odors. They had to take doses of only 12 grams daily. By taking brewer's yeast and desiccated liver plus natural vitamin C (rose hips, etc.), there would gradually develop a condition inhospitable to an oversupply of cholesterol in the arteries, and it would be effected by natural vitamins.

It seems that pyridoxine is also involved in the process by which the body uses fat. In *The Journal of Chronic Diseases* for July, 1955, there is an article called "Is Atherosclerosis a Condition of Pyridoxal Deficiency?" written by Henry A. Schroeder, M.D., whose studies on the relationship of environment to heart disease we have reported in an earlier chapter. Dr. Schroeder tells us that too little pyridoxine in the diet of monkeys produces in general the same condition as human hardening of the arteries. He says also that a deficiency of pyridoxine in rats causes high blood pressure. There is evidence, he says, that the whole process takes place in the blood vessels of these animals very much as it does in those of man.

Dr. Schroeder gives us an excellent estimate of the amount of pyridoxine in the average American diet. About half the pyridoxine in grain is lost when the grain is processed. Canned vegetables contain little, although fresh vegetables and fruits are quite rich in it. The processing of milk and meat and the cooking of food result in substantial losses of the vitamin. Any amount of heat or light, damages pyridoxine.

It is estimated that an adult may need from two

to three milligrams of pyridoxine daily. Losses after processing and cooking may make it impossible for us to get enough of the vitamin, especially during winter.

"Therefore from the incomplete data in the literature, it is entirely possible that the American adult is maintained on a marginal intake of this important coenzyme (pyridoxine) during periods of the year in which fresh vegetables and fruits are not available and processed foods and meats are widely used." Of course, too, one must take into account the quite considerable group of people who simply do not eat fresh raw fruits and vegetables even when they are available. Such folks would be bound to be lacking in pyridoxine the year round.

Now for the part pyridoxine plays in fat metabolism. Part of its job is to assist the body in using the unsaturated fatty acids—those important kinds of fat which occur in unhydrogenated vegetable oils and not in animal fats to any great extent. If there were a shortage of these unsaturated fats in the diet, one might need even more of the B vitamin pyridoxine than otherwise; if there were plenty of these fats in the diet, then one might need less pyridoxine. The American diet is notoriously lacking in liquid vegetable and cereal oils, especially as compared to other countries where little animal fat is eaten and liquid oils are used exclusively for cooking and for baking. We know that cholesterol, the fatty substance that collects on artery walls in hardening of the arteries, is dissolved by the unsaturated fatty acids. Dr. Schroeder also tells us that the cholesterol levels in the blood of monkeys deficient in pyridoxine is higher than that of monkeys which are getting plenty of the vitamin, which seems to indicate that pyridoxine plays a part, too, in the whole complicated business of how the body uses fats—for good or for harm.

Pyridoxine as well as choline can be assured through adequate supplies of brewer's yeast, desiccated liver and blackstrap molasses. It also comes in raw fruits and vegetables, in heart, wheat germ and peanuts.

Inositol

According to many independent medical observers, inositol, another fragment of the vitamin B complex, is concerned in some way with the metabolism of fat, as well as cholesterol. There have been numerous researches on animals as well as on people that have proven that the daily taking of the vitamin inositol will result in a lowering of the cholesterol content of the blood.

An article in *Newsweek* for September 11, 1950, describes the experiments of Dr. Louis B. Dotti, Dr. William C. Felch and Miss Stephanie J. Ilka of St. Luke's Hospital, New York, who experimented with feeding two groups of rabbits a capsule of cholesterol daily. One group of rabbits received just cholesterol and a regulation diet. The other group of rabbits got, in addition to the cholesterol, a capsule of inositol. At the end of the feeding period the first group of rabbits showed an increase of 337 percent in the cholesterol content of their blood. Those who had received inositol, too, showed an increase of only 181 percent.

This same group of researchers (Felch and Dotti) in the *Proceedings of the Society of Experimental Biology and Medicine* (72: 376, 1949) describes the effect of inositol on a group of 30 diabetic patients over an 8-week period which resulted in a marked decrease in the blood of cholesterol. In a booklet of the Mellon Institute called *The Biochemistry of Inositol* there is an entire chapter with many medical references describing the effect of inositol in lowering blood cholesterol levels. There can be no question that this vitamin is an effective agent in preventing cholesterol from attaining dangerous proportions in the blood.

We have already discussed Dr. Yudkin's findings that refined white sugar is bad news for the circulatory system. But, in addition to Yudkin's findings, it is now known that the practice of eating sugar results in robbing the body of its vitamin B_1 (called thiamin). Thiamin is one of the most important vitamins for good health. It is necessary for growth, good appetite and smooth functioning of the digestive tract. It plays so big a part in nerve health that it is called the "morale" vitamin. Most important of all, thiamin is vitally concerned with the digestion and assimilation of all carbohydrate foods—the sugars and starches. It must be present in considerable quantity if these foods are to be used at all by the body.

Thiamin is stolen from our bodies by these robber foods—white sugar, synthetic sugar, white flour, prepared cereals and many other refined and processed foods. If you eat carbohydrates in natural forms you do not experience any thiamin deficiency because the thiamin to digest the sugar or starch is present in the natural food. For instance, blackstrap molasses contains a great deal of natural sugar. It also has thiamin and a number of the other B vitamins, ready to go to work. Refined white sugar is the product that remains after all these B vitamins as well as many other valuable minerals have been removed from the molasses. When you eat white sugar in coffee, cakes, candies, pies, ice cream and soft drinks, you are presenting your digestive tract with large quantities of sugar to be digested and no thiamin or other B vitamins to aid in the process. In order to handle this sugar at all, the body must steal thiamin from other processes and from its storage places in the liver, kidney and heart. This means that if you eat much white sugar, if you eat some of it every day, you are almost bound to suffer from thiamin deficiency. If you are a heart case such dietary habit is cold suicide. We might express it thus: Sugar equals vitamin B deficiency equals heart trouble.

Now let us proceed into a discussion of the medical writings which show the relationship between heart trouble and vitamin B deficiency. In a book called *The Avitaminoses* by Walter H. Eddy, Ph.D., and Gilbert Doldorf, M.D. (published by The Williams & Wilkins Company), appears the statement, "Thiamin deficiency impairs the function of the heart, increases the tendency to extravascular fluid collections and results in terminal cardiac standstill." The authors show how the famous English research physician, Sir Robert McCarrison, in experiments with pigeons, produced cardiac (heart) changes in them by feeding them a vitamin B deficient diet. Eddy and Doldorf describe another experiment in which congestive heart failure was produced in pigeons and then cured by thiamin.

In the book *Nutrition and Diet in Health and Disease* by James S. McLester, M.D. (W. B. Saunders Company), it is stated that a thiamin deficiency causes a degeneration in the heart muscles. Pigs that were fed a thiamin-free diet showed a scarring in the right side of the heart.

F. V. McCollum, Ph.D., Sc.D., LL.D., in *The Newer Knowledge of Nutrition* (The Macmillan Company), shows that the normal heart rate of the rat is 500 to 550 beats per minute but when they are fed a diet low in thiamin for about three weeks the rate goes down to about 350 per minute. In fact this reduction is so dependable an occurrence on lowering the thiamin intake that it is used in laboratories to test the thiamin content of certain vitamin products. McCollum states that where the heart rate of deficient animals went down, it could be brought up again automatically within four hours after the administration of thiamin.

In the book *Vitaminology* by Walter H. Eddy, M.D., (Williams and Wilkins), the fact is discussed that a thiamin deficiency leads to beriberi disease. He says, "A definite relation of thiamin deficiency to cardiac function has long been recognized. . . . The characteristics of beriberi heart in human subjects are enlargement (usually of the right side), decreased circulation time, elevated or subnormal venous pressure, less difference than normal between the oxygen content of arterial and venous blood, and usually rapid recovery following thiamin therapy. Similar effects are observed in patients developing thiamin deficiency through the excessive use of alcohol. In both these cases the heart is tremendously dilated and the edema (swelling) is massive." This book is just chock full of instances of heart damage where the thiamin in the diet is lowered, but there is one statement that is extremely significant: "The effect of thiamin was interpreted as increasing arterial tone."

In the *New Zealand Medical Journal* for June, 1952, there is an article by G. L. Brinkman, M.D., in which four unfamiliar forms of heart failure are described due to faulty nutrition mostly due to a lack of thiamin.

There are other parts of the vitamin B complex which should also be considered in the treatment of this subject. For example—biotin. A deficiency of biotin produced symptoms of lassitude, sleepiness, muscular pains, loss of appetite, pallor, dryness of skin, disturbances of the nervous system and a feeling of distress in the region of the heart.

In our later discussion of vitamin C, we will show how it is a factor in fortifying the body against conditions of stress. There seems to be evidence also that vitamin B serves the same purpose. The B fractions which are so involved include pantothenic acid, riboflavin, folic acid and vitamin B_{12} as well as our old friend thiamin. There is a specific site of trouble—the adrenal glands—involved when vitamin deficiency reduced the ability to withstand stress.

Investigators have found that rats on a diet deficient in pantothenic acid showed an inability of the white blood cells to withstand stress. There is a considerable amount of animal experimental data which proves conclusively that both vitamin B and vitamin C factors enable the body to withstand tension-caused illness.

The consumption of sugar and alcohol rob the body of vitamin B. There are other practices that do the same thing. White flour, prepared cereals and many other refined foods are serious offenders in this regard, because the vitamin B that has been removed is badly needed to aid the digestion of carbohydrates.

Sleeping pills should not be taken, for the same reason. The barbiturates block the progress of carbohydrate metabolism and so add to the difficulty of securing enough thiamin.

Raw fish is another thief of thiamin. Dr. Eddy in his book *Vitaminology* tells us that 100 grams of raw clams contain enough anti-thiamin enzyme to destroy 7 1/2 milligrams of thiamin. This astonishing fact about raw seafood was discovered on a fox ranch in Minnesota where the foxes were falling ill from a disease that looked like thiamin deficiency, one-tenth of their diet consisting of raw fish. Cooking the fish completely eradicated the illness. Remember, therefore, that raw clams and oysters are brigands and steal large quantities of our limited store of vitamin B. It is interesting to note that the Japanese who are great raw fish and polished-rice eaters, do not have a high longevity rate.

Estrogen, a hormone administered in certain diseases, especially where individuals are inclined to be deficient in the B vitamins, will greatly cut down three of the B complexes—thiamin, riboflavin and niacin.

The sulfa drugs are mentioned in all literature dealing with vitamin enemies. Some of the B vitamins are manufactured in our intestines, so that, even if our diet is lacking in B vitamins, we may still get by, so long as the friendly "intestinal flora" go on producing B vitamins for us. The sulfa drugs upset this whole machinery and, if given long enough, they cut off this supply of vitamins. This is why pneumonia patients, for instance, whose doctors give them large doses of sulfa drugs may recover almost miraculously from the disease, but find that they are left in a state of terrible depression, fatigue and digestive disorder which may go on for years until they catch up on the necessary supply of B vitamins.

We can see, therefore, that if we assure ourselves sufficient vitamin B, preferably in the form of supplements to the regular diet, such as brewer's yeast, desiccated liver, wheat germ and blackstrap molasses, we will be moving in the right direction towards preventing an undue accumulation of fatty deposits in the artery walls.

Another element which can help guard you against heart attack is pangamic acid, also known as vitamin B_{15}. While not yet available as a pharmaceutical, this vitamin holds forth great promise as an important weapon in the fight against hypoxia (lack of oxygen).

Good results have been reported with B_{15} in the treatment of rheumatic heart disease. arteriosclerosis and angina pectoris. According to impressive evidence compiled in many European countries where it is available, this vitamin offers life-saving opportunities for the actual prevention of atherosclerosis.

Think of pangamic acid as "instant oxygen," and you will understand its lifesaving potential. Its direct action, a Russian scientific team explains, is to stimulate the hypophysis of the suprarenal glands. The hypophysis is a kind of bump located on the glands above the kidneys which have an important detoxifying function. By stimulating this activity, pangamic acid retards the accumulation of toxic waste that results from an insufficiency of oxygen. Thus the hypoxia does less damage and a longer period of time remains for normal oxygen metabolism to be re-established without damage to the organism.

When you consider that it is lack of oxygen that snuffs out the spark of life when there is a heart attack, you can readily understand how important any substance which conserves oxygen can be.

The value of a food substance that actually permits the body to function well on reduced oxygen intake is immeasurable. To be well stocked with this vitamin could mean the difference between life and death, between escaping a heart attack or the sudden death of cardiac arrest. Beef heart is the best natural source of vitamin B_{15}.

The condemned anti-cholesterol drug, MER/29, was used by at least 400,000 patients before the government blew the whistle on it as a cause of blindness, falling hair, skin disease and a loss of sexual desire. This mass exposure to a harmful drug is the more unforgivable when one considers that a harmless vitamin could have been prescribed instead: nicotinic acid, a B vitamin, known to be more effective and safer than MER/29 or any other drug used to cut cholesterol. But doctors rarely use a vitamin when a drug is available to treat the same thing, and they didn't use nicotinic acid very much.

Laymen find this hard to understand since nicotinic acid, according to reports by a number of investigators, is at least as effective against cholesterol as any dangerous drug. Dr. William B. Parsons, Jr., director of research at the Jackson Clinic and Foundation, Madison, Wisconsin, has been urging that a major long-range test be given to nicotinic acid therapy in control of high cholesterol to settle once and for all its superiority in the field. A study to be supported by the National Institutes of Health, planned as early as March, 1961, has yet to be begun.

Doctors are amazingly consistent in their concern about side effects where *nutrients* are used in medicinal doses. Mention a vitamin or a mineral as a treatment for disease, and physicians become terribly concerned about the possibility of flushing, loose stool, mild nausea, etc. They would rather risk liver damage, cataract, serious skin disease or even cancer from a drug sold by a big-name manufacturer than take a chance on a vitamin.

Dr. Parsons demonstrates this attitude: "Doctors keep asking me, 'Isn't there an awful flush?' The so-called flush consists of a warm feeling, accompanied by a redness of the face and upper part of the body that lasts for twenty minutes to half an hour after each large dose of nicotinic acid early in the treatment. This effect usually disappears after the first few days on the treatment, and few of the patients are ever concerned enough to make more than a passing reference to it. Compared with the effect from almost any commercial drug compound, it is negligible."

In a test with 90 patients doctors found that a "significant minority" developed changes in the liver enzyme function test after long-term therapy. When the patients were studied more closely, the abnormal liver tests were shown due to the synthetic *aluminum* nicotinate only, and this side-effect was eliminated when the medication was stopped, or when *plain nicotinic acid was substituted* in the same dosage. Nausea has shown up, but again it was because aluminum nicotinate was used in place of simple nicotinic acid. Dr. Parsons said even the aluminum nicotinate side reactions are minor and should not discourage investigators from using it. But apparently plain nicotinic acid is even better.

Medical Tribune reported early studies at the University of Saskatchewan where Drs. Altschul, Hoffer and Stephen lowered cholesterol concentrations in rabbits as well as in humans with nicotinic acid. In several cases visible cholesterol deposits (in skin or in tendons) were eliminated by nicotinic acid, and results were achieved in periods ranging from a few months to a year or so.

Essential to the function of the liver where part of blood manufacture takes place, folic acid, another B-complex vitamin, has come to be recognized for its therapeutic effect on anemias and in the treatment of sprue. Recent use in the treatment of arteriosclerosis opens dramatic new possibilities for the people over 40 who are suffering the slowdown of the debilitating condition commonly known as "hardening of the arteries."

Such is the conclusion put forth by Dr. Tibor L. Kopjas in an article in the *Journal of the American Geriatric Society* (November, 1966) on the "Effect of Folic Acid on Collateral Circulation in Diffuse Chronic Arteriosclerosis."

Since folic acid seemed to be an effective dilator for small arteries, Dr. Kopjas was intrigued with its possible potential in the treatment of diffuse chronic arteriosclerosis where the small arteries are called upon to play a vital role. He undertook a study of 17 patients whom he divided into three groups according to age, duration of disease, and the degree of arterial damage.

In the first group, folic acid was administered intravenously to determine its immediate effects on the small arteries. About 40 minutes after the injection, persons in this group, who were already suffering impaired vision as a result of insufficient circulation to the eyes (and extremities), showed marked improvement and were able to read two lines below the lines recorded before medication.

Group two was made up of seven patients who had had chronic diffuse peripheral vascular disease for at least ten years. Most of them responded well to the folic acid. After the injection, all experienced the manifestations of improved circulation —pleasant warm feelings in the face and head within five minutes, in the hands within ten minutes.

Six patients comprising group three had diabetes mellitus, with diabetic retinopathy, where eyesight is greatly diminished, and arteriosclerosis obliterans (almost complete roadblock). Each took a 5 mg. folic acid tablet daily for four weeks. Improvement in vision and in skin temperature of affected limbs was observed by four patients. In two of these cases, there was healing of pregangrenous toe ulcers—dramatic manifestation of improved circulation. At no time did Dr. Kopjas note any increase in blood pressure or pulse rates. There were no side effects either during or after the study.

Those who are still relying on multi-purpose synthetic vitamin formulas may be getting none, or at best an insufficient dosage, of folic acid. While a regulation, issued by the FDA in 1960, restricted the daily dose in vitamin preparations to no more than .4 mg. except on a prescription-only basis, we have been able to find in the *Physician's Desk Reference* very few multi-vitamin preparations with any folic acid content at all.

Manifestations of folic acid deficiency include cramps, pain, weakness and numbness of the feet, legs and hands. If you are suffering any of these conditions, you would be wise to take stock of your nutrition. Natural vegetable sources are green leafy vegetables—lettuce, spinach, endive. Other vegetables with folic acid content are blackeyed peas, carrots, mushrooms, cauliflower and broccoli. Among the fruits, watermelon, cantaloupe, tomatoes and oranges are relatively high. Wheat germ is a good source, but other cereals are either only moderately good or poor sources. Liver is an excellent source but muscle meats are poor to fair. Beef and pork loin may contain only 1/6 to 1/10 as much as spinach on a dry weight basis. Cow's milk has practically no folic acid. Mother's milk is a good source when the mother's intake is adequate.

An adequate supply of vitamin C is absolutely necessary if folic acid is not to be destroyed by antagonists present in the body—antagonists which may account for the anemia or scurvy. Biotin, too, is in some way involved in folic acid metabolism. In fact, one cannot devise a natural diet so deficient in one vitamin as to produce disease and still be adequate in the others. Dr. Tom Spies, after a ten-year study of synthetic folic acid published in *General Practitioner,* August, 1957, deplored the effort expended by gifted physicians who don't understand that "nutritive failure" is not the failure of a single vitamin.

In fact, while folic acid is a nutrient essential for life and is widely distributed in nature, if one subsists on processed and canned foods, it is easy to develop a deficiency. The research study by Dr. Kopjas, pointing to this vitamin as an important element in the therapeutic treatment of arteriosclerosis, may well indicate that diets rich in this element could help to cut down on the incidence of one of modern society's great tragedies, the "sudden death" caused by cardiovascular complications.

Lecithin for Your Arteries

In treating patients for high cholesterol content of the blood, many physicians advise cutting out all foods that are high in cholesterol. This would include: brains, egg yolk, fish roe, kidney, liver, sweetbreads—foods especially high in cholesterol.

Now these are all good foods, containing vitamins and minerals that we need. How can we possibly cure a sick person by taking away the very foods that will give him large amounts of vitamin A, the B vitamins, vitamin E and the unsaturated fatty acids, sometimes called vitamin F? The sick person needs these vitamins even more than the well person. So, even though we may reduce the cholesterol content of his blood by removing foods that are high in cholesterol, we may also bring on something far worse if we consistently deprive him of the foods he needs.

A far better approach is to study everything about the patient's diet and see if perhaps he is getting too little of something else which is the very thing he needs so that his body can use cholesterol properly and it will not accumulate in his blood vessels or gall bladder. Is there such a substance? A great many medical researchers believe there is and they have years of hard work to prove their theories.

The substance that apparently protects against accumulations of cholesterol is lecithin. It is pronounced *less-i-thin* with the accent on the first syllable. The word comes from the Greek *Likithos,* meaning *the yolk of an egg.* For lecithin is most abundant in egg yolk. In fact, when it was first studied in Germany towards the end of the last century, the researchers could then obtain lecithin only from egg yolk and this was too expensive a source for use by the general public. So they didn't get very far with their research and it was not until quite recently that another source, soybeans, has been discovered.

How does it happen that the lecithin occurs in egg yolk where cholesterol also is plentiful? Doesn't it sound like another of Mother Nature's provisions for good health? Cholesterol without lecithin can be harmful. So they are both included in this one especially healthful food. Why then should we have any trouble with cholesterol —aren't we all getting enough lecithin in our food?

Apparently not. The processing which our various fats and oils go through before they appear on grocery shelves destroys the lecithin content, but leaves the cholesterol. Hydrogenated fats, for instance,—the shortenings used in pastry and for frying—do not contain lecithin, for it has been destroyed in the hydrogenation process. What happens as a result? The lecithin was put there by nature to act as an emulsifying agent for the cholesterol.

This means simply that when the cholesterol tends to coalesce or lump together, the lecithin breaks it up, mixes with it, and keeps it finely divided so that it can be circulated throughout the body as a perfectly stable "emulsion" that will not solidify or congeal. Once the lecithin is removed, there is nothing to keep the cholesterol moving along through the bloodstream—it cakes; it gathers in lumps.

H. D. Keston and R. Silbowitz reported in the *Proceedings of the Society of Experimental Biology and Medicine,* volume 49, 1942, that feeding lecithin to rabbits who were receiving large amounts of cholesterol kept the cholesterol from collecting in the blood and in the blood vessels and prevented hardening of the arteries in the rabbits. G. L. Duff and T. P. B. Payne wrote in the *Journal of Experimental Medicine,* volume 92, 1950, that they had showed in laboratory animals that the amount of cholesterol taken is *not* the important thing in hardening of the arteries—*the important thing is the instability* of the cholesterol. That is, when the cholesterol is not emulsified, it deposits on artery walls. Lecithin, of course, emulsifies it.

D. Adlersburg and H. Sobotka showed in *Gastroenterology,* volume 1, 1943, that lecithin helps greatly in absorbing vitamin A and fats in patients whose diseases make this nearly impossible. A. Scharf and C. A. Slanetz tell us that there is an unknown factor in lecithin which is absolutely essential for the body in order to use vitamin A properly. It also improves the utilization of vitamin E in their laboratory experiments. This information comes from the *Proceedings of the Society of Experimental Biology and Medicine*, volume 57, 1944.

Seeds, as well as egg yolks and soybeans, are a rich source of lecithin. Primitive peoples eat seeds of all kinds—melon seeds, sunflower seeds, cereal seeds, corn kernels, acorns, millet, whole rice and so forth. But what seeds does the average American ever eat that have not been tampered with? Nuts are the only ones we can think of at the moment and even these he seems unable to eat unless they have been roasted to nothingness.

If you are worried about hardening of the arteries—and who of us over the age of 40 is not?—your best bet is to include lecithin in your food supplements, *especially* if you cannot possibly omit from your meals all the processed foods which will increase your cholesterol without increasing your lecithin.

Lecithin for human consumption is made chiefly from soybeans. In fact, soya-lecithin has come to be the name generally used for lecithin because it is practically always made from soybeans. The way soya-lecithin was discovered is typical of our modern blundering way of doing things. Soybeans have become a profitable crop in this country, and the oil they contain is used for all kinds of different products, most of them having nothing to do with food—rubber, petroleum, paint, ink, leather, soap, shaving creams, putty and so forth. So, as the chemists were devising ways and means of using this perfectly splendid food to manufacture these various non-food articles, they found that one substance interfered with many of the processes they wanted to use. So they removed the substance—lecithin. It became a waste product.

Isn't that a typical feat of modern genius—to remove from a food product the main substance that makes it valuable as food and then sit and ponder what to do with it so it won't be wasted! Lecithin is used in some food processing, for it is a good emulsifier outside the body as well as inside. But it apparently never occurred to anybody that it was put into soybeans for some nutritional purpose, and certainly it would never occur to anybody to put it *back* into foods so that they would be more nourishing! In our country today the food industry seems bent on making food just something that will last a long time on grocery shelves, will look pretty and will be convenient. And of course all of this means that more and more nutritional value must be sacrificed.

Take lecithin—it's convenient, inexpensive and easy to take—if you have the slightest suspicion that you are getting too much cholesterol for your own good. Don't cut down on eggs and butter—but do cut down on the processed foods from which the lecithin has been removed!

Rutin for Vascular Disorders

A recent subject for investigation in cases of hypertension has been rutin—a substance found most plentifully in buckwheat. Rutin is a part of vitamin P. Apparently vitamin P, like the other vitamins, has many parts called "flavones." All of them are more or less related and have many of the same properties so far as human health is concerned, but some parts appear to be more effective in the treatment of certain disorders.

High blood pressure brings with it certain dangers, not the least of which is hemorrhage—including cerebral hemorrhage which we speak of as a "stroke." In cases of stroke, the small blood vessels or capillaries rupture, due to the pressure upon them, and the hemorrhaging of the blood from this ruptured vessel brings about the unconsciousness and other symptoms of stroke as "cerebral accidents."

It would seem that more is involved in this rupturing of a blood vessel than just the pressure being put on it by the blood. Perhaps, researchers have reasoned, part of the fault may lie in the weakness of the actual walls of the blood vessels, or capillary fragility. Interest in rutin was aroused by the discovery that apparently it had a lot to do with maintaining the walls of the blood vessels so that they do not become fragile and hence are less likely to rupture and cause serious illness or death.

Immediately, a whole series of problems in research presented themselves. First of all, how can the fragility of the blood vessels be measured? It is relative to the blood pressure of course, and the higher the blood pressure goes, the more hardy the vessels must be not to rupture. In a patient suffering from stroke, one may assume that perhaps his blood vessels were indeed fragile, but how can one discover this *before* the accident takes place so that the patient can be treated for fragile blood vessels and so perhaps never have a stroke? The problem of measuring the fragility of blood vessels has never actually been solved satisfactorily, and this is one reason for the doubt and confusion around the whole subject of rutin for high blood pressure patients.

Working with laboratory animals, there are several methods of measuring fragility of capillaries. H. K. Hellerstein, M.D., and his colleagues at several hospitals in Illinois and Ohio experimented by producing in animals blood pressure high enough to cause hemorrhaging from the blood vessels. To one group of animals they gave rutin ten days before inducing the high blood pressure. Another group received no rutin. As reported in *The American Heart Journal* for August, 1951, all of the animals died as a result of the high blood pressure, but those which received rutin did not show any evidence of hemorrhaging as the other animals did.

In humans, direct observation of the capillaries, as we mentioned in an earlier chapter, can be made in the eyes—and only in the eyes. These capillaries are examined carefully every time you see your eye specialist, the ophthalmologist. An extremely interesting article on the use of rutin, by

Dr. L. B. Somerville-Large, appeared in the *Transactions of the Ophthalmological Society of the United Kingdom,* volume 69, 1949-1950. Dr. Somerville-Large states that "in the eye we have what appears to be the only opportunity the human body affords of actually observing lesions (disorders) associated with capillary dysfunction. We must, therefore, forgive our medical colleagues for their caution in recognizing the value of rutin."

He says that the commonest conditions in which the capillaries seem to be out of order are diabetes, toxic and inflammatory conditions, high blood pressure and hardening of the arteries. Although hypertension of itself has no relation to capillary fragility, he says, six to ten percent of those hypertensives who do have increased capillary fragility suffer from hemorrhages in the retina of the eye, and cerebral or brain hemorrhages. He gives doses of two 60-milligram tablets of rutin three times a day making a total dosage of 360 milligrams daily. "I find," says he, "that the larger doses give a more rapid and more complete negative result to capillary fragility tests." Incidentally, he always combines the rutin with 200 milligrams of vitamin C daily.

It is interesting to note that throughout the discussion of vitamin P and rutin in medical literature, it is suggested that vitamin P and vitamin C work closely together, and better results are always obtained when they are given together. Note, too, that Dr. Somerville-Large gives quite a large dose of vitamin C—200 milligrams. At the present time the official recommendation for the minimum daily intake of vitamin C is only 70 milligrams and it is believed that most of us don't even get that much! Does it not seem reasonable that two or three times this amount of vitamin C every day might do a lot to prevent the capillary fragility which is responsible for so much distress today? Remember that vitamin C is also involved in keeping the intercellular membranes healthy.

In conclusion, Dr. Somerville-Large states that in his experience he has not yet "met a case in which the capillary fragility skin test has not been reduced with rutin to well within normal limits." In speaking of the length of time it is necessary to continue taking the rutin, he says, "To me at the present time it looks like a life sentence. Whenever rutin has been discontinued the capillary fragility has again increased. Also if the rutin is discontinued and the vitamin C alone persisted with, again the capillary fragility increases."

Another example of the use of rutin in treating capillary fragility is presented by Bicknell and Prescott in *Vitamins in Medicine.* The authors tell of 12 children in a group of 100 allergic children who were treated with 100 to 150 milligrams of vitamin P daily for six months. At the end of this time their capillary resistance became normal.

What application can we make of all these experiences to our daily life? First of all, if vitamin P (of which rutin is a part), is really a vitamin, how much of it do we perhaps need every day? The Federation of the American Societies for Experimental Biology has voted to discontinue the use of the term "vitamin" in relation to vitamin P. They declare that it has not been proved as yet that these substances (the flavones) are essential to good health and that their absence in diet will cause any disorder that can be cured by administering them. However, people in other countries, and this country as well, go right on calling the flavones "vitamin P." Bicknell and Prescott state that the daily requirement may be not less than 33 units daily "and possibly considerably more."

Just like vitamin C, vitamin P is destroyed by cooking in an open vessel. So, much of the vitamin P value of foods is lost in cooking. Once again we are faced with the absolute necessity for eating plenty of fresh raw fruits and vegetables, for it is in these that vitamin P is found in the largest amounts, along with vitamin C. The rutin concentrate used by doctors in treating hypertensive patients is made from buckwheat. Rutin occurs chiefly in the leaves of buckwheat which may contain as much as seven or eight percent of rutin. It is rapidly destroyed when the leaves are dried slowly, so they must be processed with the greatest care. After the leaves are completely dried, there seems to be no further loss of rutin.

If you are suffering from high blood pressure and your doctor advises taking rutin to avoid any possibility of a stroke, we would certainly go along with his advice, on the basis of the evidence we have collected. If you are perfectly healthy and interested in preserving the state of your blood vessels so that you will not suffer from these disorders later on, then by all means see that you get, every day, plenty of foods in which vitamin P (hence rutin) occurs, along with vitamin C.

Here is a list of foods that are rich in vitamin P and we have given you their vitamin C content as well. We hope you notice that, just as rose hips are many, many times richer in vitamin C than any other food, so too they are especially rich in vitamin P.

Foods with High Vitamin P Content

	Vitamin P Content in Units	*Vitamin C Content in Milligrams*
Apricot	75-100 in 8 apricots	4
Blackberry	60-100 in 3/4 cup	3
Black Currant	200-500 in 1 cup	150
Cabbage (summer)	100 in 1 cup, raw	50
Cherry, Black	60-100 in 12 large cherries	12
Grape, Black	500-1000 in 1 small bunch	3
Grape, White	500-1000 in 1 small bunch	4
Grapefruit	100 in 1/2 grapefruit	45
Lemon Juice	450-750 in 8 tablespoons	25
Orange	300-500 in 1 medium orange	50
Parsley	130 in 1 cup	70
Plum	50-200 in 3 medium plums	5
Prune	300-400 in 8 medium prunes	4
Rose Hips	240-680 in 100 grams	500 to 6000

Vitamin K Necessary for Blood Clotting

Lack of vitamin K may be the prime factor with cardiovascular diseases related to uncontrolled bleeding. The most common of these is stroke caused by the hemorrhaging of an artery in the brain. Surgery and childbirth also require that the blood be capable of clotting adequately or complications may result.

Vitamin K helps to form prothrombin, a substance that promotes blood clotting—but the liver must be functioning properly or some of the vitamin K absorbed will not be utilized adequately. Gallstones or liver disease may inhibit bile flow and interfere with absorption of the fat soluble vitamin K. Diarrhea and colitis may damage the absorptive surfaces of the small intestines, again preventing full usage of vitamin K. For people who unknowingly suffer from liver or intestinal effects, the need for vitamin K is all the more serious.

Natural vitamin K can be supplied by pork liver, fish meal, egg yolk, leafy green vegetables, tomatoes, wheat germ, soybeans and potatoes. When these foods are not included in the diet for a period of time, our blood clotting ability may be seriously impaired.

A study by John Udall, M.D., of the Maricopa County General Hospital in Phoenix, Arizona, appears in the *Journal of the American Medical Association* (October 11, 1965). He found that when healthy volunteers ate nothing but polished rice, black coffee, granulated sugar, and a multi-vitamin tablet (without vitamin K) for three weeks, blood-clotting time rose from 14.8 seconds to 16.0 seconds. When pork liver and fresh spinach were added, one man showed "three sharp falls in prothrombin time, almost to normal." Dr. Udall concluded, "Foods, rather than bacterial synthesis, probably provide most vitamin K for humans."

Dietary vitamin K also seems to play a role in the prevention of heart disease. Writing in the *Tri-State Medical Journal* (February, 1959), Hunter McGuire Doles mentions that Negroes in the southern United States, where home-grown vegetables are an economic necessity, have lower rates of coronary thrombosis than the whites. A high vegetable diet also seems to account for the "extremely rare" incidences of coronary thrombosis in East Africa and myocardial infarction (blockage of heart muscle) in West Africa.

The *Journal of the American Medical Association* (March 14, 1964) reports a study in which heart patients, who had been treated with anti-coagulant drugs (to prevent clots), also ate high amounts of spinach and other green vegetables for two weeks. Their "free prothrombin returned to normal," and prothrombin time decreased. The dangers of the anticoagulants had been eliminated.

Vitamin C and the Blood Vessels

There may be vitamins of which it can be assumed that just about everything important to know about them has already been learned. Vitamin C is not one of that group, however. Although it was identified in pure crystalline form as ascorbic acid 35 years ago, and has been studied intensively ever since, it seems that our knowledge of the many functions of this fantastic nutrient is only at its beginning. Hardly a month goes by that we do not learn something new about the seemingly endless variety of functions, all fundamentally important to health, that are performed by this one vitamin.

One of the more recent discoveries about vitamin C concerns its role in preventing protracted bleeding. Writing in *The Lancet* (May 6, 1967), Drs. G. P. McNicol and A. S. Douglas, of the University of Glasgow Department of Medicine, reported their experience in two interesting cases.

The first case concerned a 55-year-old man who, after a minor injury to his right leg, developed extensive bruising. "A few days after the injury and bruising of the right leg, spontaneous bruising of the left leg developed. His diet consisted of white bread, tea sardines, an occasional slice of meat and an occasional egg. He disliked fruit and vegetables and had not eaten any of these for at least two years."

Such a spontaneous appearance of bruises indicates to a doctor the hemorrhaging of the capillaries, which is related to a failure of the clotting mechanism. A blood analysis was ordered and it was found that "platelet adhesiveness was abnormally low."

As we described earlier, the platelets are microscopic circular or oval discs which are found in the blood in large quantity. They are an integral factor in the ability of blood to coagulate, a function which they influence by possessing a stickiness which causes them to clump together wherever the blood flows out of a vessel.

"The patient was maintained on a hospital diet for two days without ascorbic acid supplement. A second blood sample was then obtained which showed adhesiveness essentially unchanged. Ascorbic acid was then administered in a dosage of 700 milligrams per day. No new scorbutic lesions developed thereafter and the existing manifestations disappeared rapidly. . . . After the administration of ascorbic acid, platelet adhesiveness rapidly increased to a high level, at which it was maintained."

The second patient, a woman of 61, showed a similar lack of adhesiveness in her platelets with the blood consequently being unable to clot properly. And she also responded quickly to the administration of vitamin C.

In their discussion of the meaning of their report, Drs. McNicol and Douglas point out that although acquired hemorrhagic disease has been recognized for at least seven centuries as a symptom of scurvy, there have been very few reports of abnormalities in the blood that can be identified in a laboratory as a clinical sign of vitamin C deficiency. "We describe here a newly-defined abnormality, decreased platelet adhesiveness. . . ."

Of course it is only the ability to define the abnormality that is new. Loss of stickiness of the platelets through a deficiency of vitamin C has undoubtedly been going on as long as human beings have had to subsist on diets that did not contain enough of this vitamin. But the ability to define, now, just what it is that happens to the blood that causes hemorrhaging when there is insufficient vitamin C represents a definite step forward. It now becomes apparent that many cases of clotting slowness or complete inability to clot may have a definite though hitherto unguessed connection to the vitamin C levels of the blood. And it seems likely that soon we will be reading new reports of how previously untreatable types of hemorrhage have been treated by the administration of vitamin C.

To the hundred reasons why we all need plenty of vitamin C every single day there has thus been added one more. And this, we are convinced, is only the beginning. The more we learn about this vitamin, the more we are convinced that there is literally no end to the number of ways in which it aids health.

If it is true, as most doctors believe, that a man is as old as his arteries, then there is no reason ever to grow old in the biological sense if you get enough vitamin C in your diet. Such is the clear conclusion to be derived from an article in the *Journal of the American Geriatrics Society* (December, 1966) on "Aging, Atherosclerosis and Ascorbic

Acid Metabolism." Coming from the Southern Bio-Research Institute of Lakeland, Florida, the lengthy report and survey was written by Boris Sokoloff, M.D., Ph.D., director of the Institute, with four associates. It consists of both experimental evidence and widespread corroboration from the medical literature that ascorbic acid (vitamin C) is the key element in averting atherosclerosis and that, in fact, atherosclerosis may well be a vitamin C deficiency disease.

The mechanism that is described by Dr. Sokoloff and associates as the manner in which atherosclerosis is caused is a rather complicated one, but one that we feel is worth the reader's efforts to understand. In the first place, the authors point out that, after many years of trying to establish a cause and effect relationship between cholesterol and the clogging of the arteries with fatty deposits (atherosclerosis), leading research scientists have come to believe that it is some other element in fats, notably the triglycerides, that is the true cause.

(Incidentally, more serum triglycerides are produced by sugar than by fats. The best way to reduce triglyceride consumption, as we have mentioned earlier, is to eliminate table sugar entirely from the diet.)

What happens, then, as explained by Dr. Sokoloff, is that after a fatty and sugary meal the blood plasma becomes clogged with serum triglycerides. To combat this, the body synthesizes an enzyme known as lipoprotein lipase (LPL). Where does this LPL come from? From the walls of healthy capillaries, which directly depend on vitamin C for the maintenance of their health. Because of the action of LPL, the triglycerides are broken down into free fatty acids, along with the cholesterol, and the blood vessels are thus cleared. There is no chance for the fats to accumulate in the kind of fatty plaques that cling to the artery walls, clog them and keep the arteries themselves from receiving an adequate blood supply, so that they turn hard and brittle.

Dr. Sokoloff then goes on to cite a host of references on possible and probable reasons why, as age advances, the body should have greater difficulty in producing the LPL that is necessary to control the lipids in the bloodstream. The one that seems most significant to us is the work of a Japanese doctor, M. Higuchi, who on the basis of much experimental work concluded that there is a relationship between ascorbic acid levels and the hormone production of the sex glands. It is already known that the sex glands have a great need for vitamin C. Prostatic fluid, for example, which nourishes the sperms and keeps them alive, is extremely rich in this vitamin and must be. It is obvious that one of the effects of aging that cannot be prevented or even called abnormal is the slowing down of the activity of the sex glands. For them to cease activity entirely is never normal and would probably indicate either disease or nutritional deficiency or both. But the slowdown is inevitable.

What Higuchi uncovered is that, as the sex glands begin to decrease their level of activity, they have increasingly great needs for vitamin C in order to continue functioning at all. Higuchi concluded that the aged, particularly men, require a larger supply of ascorbic acid than do the young. Doctor Sokoloff cites half a dozen other references to validate this conclusion. And since they have this greater requirement, the sex glands will draw vitamin C away from the other tissues in order to fulfill it.

What it comes down to is that, as one grows older, the vitamin C stored in the tissues is drawn away from the capillaries to such glands as the prostate and the testicles and the adrenals as well. This leaves the capillaries less able to produce lipoprotein lipase. As a consequence, the fats in the bloodstream are not properly broken down and tend to accumulate and clog the arteries. The condition ultimately becomes atherosclerosis.

And the obvious answer, furnishing a mechanism by which it should be possible to prevent atherosclerosis, is to make sure that with every year that passes you get more vitamin C in your diet than you did the year before—substantially more. This is difficult, of course for those who try to get their vitamins entirely from food. The increase in food processing and the increasing tendency to pick fruits when they are immature so that they will store longer have both reduced the amount of vitamin C available in food. In 1960 the Department of Agriculture stated that the available vitamin C had already declined by 23 percent. By now, the decline is probably well over 30 percent.

We find it far more satisfactory to make sure of getting enough of this precious vitamin by taking daily supplements. Moreover, let us add an important word of caution.

Dr. Sokoloff, reporting his group's own experiments both on laboratory rats and on 122 patients who were kept under observation for periods from four to thirty months, points out that with regard to the blood lipids vitamin C does *not* act like a miracle drug. "Group B included 60 cases of pronounced hypercholesteremia and/or cardiac disease. In some cases the triglyceride levels were 300 milligrams per 100 ml. or higher, with low LPL activity. In 10 of the 60 cases, the beneficial effect of ascorbic acid was insignificant. In the remaining 50, improvement ranged from moderate to impressive." But while a convincingly predominant proportion were helped by vitamin C, the help in no case came overnight or even in a short period of time. Dr. Sokoloff points out that it takes five to six months before any beneficial effect whatsoever can be observed.

So if you want to help yourself prevent atherosclerosis, there is no point in waiting until trouble develops. The time to act is now, and the way to act is to obtain large amounts of vitamin C in the diet every day from now on.

Miracles with Vitamin E

"A dose of alpha tocopherol calculated by Skelton on the basis of his dog experiments and much higher than had ever been used in clinical medicine before, viz., 200 milligrams per day, was given to the patient, whose myocardial failure quickly vanished. . . . Encouraged by this I next treated my barber, who was dying from a recurrent coronary thrombosis and was in the terminal stages of heart failure with status antinosus. In three weeks' time he was playing the tympana in the local theatre. Next my mother's severe angina pectoris disappeared on alpha tocopherol therapy. Then Dr. Wilfrid Shute and I recalled our first successful angina patient of 1936 and the four other patients treated at that time. Accordingly, we began, with the assistance of Dr. Vogelsang, to collect the series of observations on cardiovascular patients that we may presume to say have changed the face of cardiology." So begins the saga of alpha tocopherol, vitamin E, as related by Dr. Evan Shute in the book, *Alpha Tocopherol in Cardiovascular Disease,* published by the Shute Foundation for Medical Research, London, Ontario, Canada.

It is an amazing story—the story told in this book—exciting, inspiring, at times heroic, but also completely scientific and objective. The Shute brothers—two physicians, Evan and Wilfrid—take the reader on a tour of their file of case histories—well over 10,000 patients treated for heart and vascular disorders with vitamin E. Of particular interest is a chapter by Dr. Wilfrid Shute on classical cardiac therapy—that is, the treatment other than vitamin E that has been used up to now for heart trouble. He discusses digitalis, quinidine, mercurial diuretics and other drugs.

He quotes the President of the Texas Heart Association who said in the *Texas State Journal of Medicine* in 1951, "When a physician makes a diagnosis of organic heart disease, he realizes that in the care of the patient he has begun a losing fight. In the earliest stages he offers general advice: 'Avoid strenuous activities; live sensibly, watch your weight; don't worry; the heart is a wonderful organ.' Before too long symptoms develop and the doctor braces the patient with digitalis or other drugs, restriction of usual activities, more rest and more encouragement. Again, before long, more urgent symptoms force a retreat. Bed rest, low sodium diet, diuretics and other well known measures are brought to the front and the line is stabilized. But not for long. All too soon increasing pressure bends the line and retreat begins again. Now there are left no more reserves—no more in the heart and no more in the hands of the one trying to help the heart. Then only surrender remains. Not infrequently the enemy strikes suddenly with overwhelming power, and surrender occurs before the doctor can mobilize his forces." How indeed could one better describe the usual case of heart disease treated by the usual methods?

This is, this *has to be,* the point of view of doctors using the time-honored prescriptions against this mysterious and deadly disease. How heart-warming and encouraging, then, to turn the page and find cheering, confident and convincing evidence of the marvelous effectiveness of vitamin E in heart and vascular cases! There are chapters in this book on the use of vitamin E in coronary sclerosis, coronary occlusion, rheumatic heart disease and hypertension. In the chapter "Tailoring the Dose" full instructions are given for using vitamin E in heart therapy, with descriptions of the various categories of patients and the characteristic problems they present in treatment.

To bring the benefits of vitamin E to laymen, science writer Herbert Bailey has written *Vitamin E: Your Key to a Healthy Heart.* This is a readable, nontechnical book for laymen in which Mr. Bailey says he is convinced that vitamin E therapy is destined to become one of the basic weapons in fighting disorders of the heart and circulatory system.

Bailey cites more than seven hundred medical researches in seventeen countries in support of his assertion. For example, Dr. V. R. O'Connor and Dr. J. P. S. Hodges of England for eight years used vitamin E in their treatment of 350 patients for conditions ranging from general arteriosclerosis to congenital heart disease. Their final conclusion (after 30 years' experience in both medicine and surgery) was that "Alpha Tocopherol (vitamin E) treatment of cardiovascular and renal diseases, as suggested by Drs. E. V. and W. E. Shute, is one of the greatest medical discoveries of the century."

In addition to many doctors, both in the United States and abroad, Bailey quotes Dr. P. L. Harris, the Director of the Department of Nutrition at the Food and Drug Administration, who is a pioneer in the pharmacologic development of vitamin E in all phases, as well as in direct experimentation on both animals and humans. Dr. Harris told Bailey: "I'm proud of my work. Conditions are changing, I believe, and vitamin E will be duly recognized as a most significant factor in human metabolism."

The noted medical author states that according to well-checked information, more than 70,000 heart-afflicted patients throughout the world have been saved or have been vastly benefited through the use of vitamin E in the last fifteen years. He cites numerous case histories and controlled studies, all carefully supervised by reputable researcher-doctor teams in seventeen countries, including the United States. He answers the puzzling question of why orthodox medical groups in America have apparently lagged far behind those of other medically advanced countries in their recognition of the new therapy.

"Perhaps the most cogent reason for the tardiness of orthodox American medical groups in accepting vitamin E's role in heart disease," Bailey says, "is that the vitamin is too versatile in its action, and most American doctors have been trained to believe that for a specific disease there must be a specific remedy." Many doctors, according to Bailey, believe that what works to heal one disease cannot possibly aid in another—or else the remedy is categorized as a cure-all or a panacea and those words are anathema to large numbers of "modern" practitioners. "Yet," Bailey states, "the fact is that it has been demonstrated, both in the laboratory and in clinical studies, that vitamin E is effective against a multitude of diseases."

Researchers during the last twenty years have shown that vitamin E (1) conserves about 50 percent of the oxygen that is ordinarily metabolized in the cells and tissues of the body. Thus the strain on the heart, and on other tissues as well is considerably reduced. (2) Vitamin E acts as a vasodilator. That is, its action allows more blood to flow through constricted arteries and veins, thereby bringing more nourishment to the heart muscles and other organs. (3) It acts as an antioxidant, slowing up the oxidative process that turns cells "rancid," and consequently delays oxygen from combining with other substances to form the deadly hydrogen peroxide, which hastens the death of a cell. This fact has been proven in tests on human beings, on animals and on tissues which have been removed from recently killed animals.

(4) Vitamin E acts as a wound healer. When used as an ingredient in an ointment at the site of a wound or burn and also when taken internally, it has been found to hasten the healing of the wound or burn—and most significantly, to reduce the amount of scar tissue in some cases. The vitamin seems to soften and dissolve the tissues that form a scar.

Bailey reports amazing results of controlled studies of vitamin E therapy on the health, strength and fertility of animals. He cites the report of the E. P. Taylor Stud Farm, which showed a 100 percent increase in profits as a direct and proven result of the benefits of the addition of vitamin E to the diet of the sires, mares and foals. One of the most striking examples of the effects of vitamin E is that of the famous race horse, Northern Dancer, whose sire and dam were fed vitamin E in appropriate doses before conception occurred and who also received equally effective doses after birth. This famous little colt was offered for sale, when a yearling, for $25,000 with no takers, and two years later had earned close to $2,000,000—having established an all-time record at the Kentucky Derby and won the Preakness. Now retired because of an injury, he has won 14 out of 17 starts and never finished out of the money.

Bailey also cites the vitamin's role in the prevention of the symptoms of old age. One of his sources is the world-famed Dr. Hans Selye of the University of Montreal, who—as we reported earlier—advances the theory that stress is the primary cause of disease and aging. In a classic experiment, Selye and his co-workers demonstrated the importance of vitamin E in the reversal as well as the prevention of the symptoms of the aging process. A group of rats was treated with chemicals that artifically induced the symptoms of old age. Another group received massive doses of vitamin E in addition to the "old age" chemicals; upon autopsy, the latter group showed no signs of premature aging. Further treatment with vitamin E actually reversed the aging process that had begun in other groups of chemically treated rats!

Vitamin E may delay the appearance of old age symptoms in man, thus possibly giving him a longer life span. A study of many mammals on earth reveals that they live to be about six times their age at maturation. Man, maturing at 25, should live to be 150 years old, by this rule of thumb.

Eighty-eight percent of American Olympic stars use wheat germ oil (an even richer source of vitamin E than wheat germ). But perhaps the most recent example of an athletic star using vitamin E is Murray Rose. who is the youngest Olympic triple gold medal winner in history. On occasions when extra muscular exertion is required, such as in swimming contests, Murray takes from 200 to 1500 international units of vitamin E along with other vitamins and minerals.

Dr. G. A. Goria of Italy, who studied many

phases of human heart action by means of an electrocardiograph, proved that vitamin E can and does improve the function of the "normal" heart as well as aiding the circulatory and metabolic processes of the body.

"In fact," says Bailey. "you can hardly name a human purpose that is not aided by large amounts of this vitamin. It is the miracle of modern medicine—unfortunately, still undiscovered by all too many."

Dr. Wilfrid Shute's own words can scarcely be improved upon in explaining how vitamin E works. They have both the ring of authenticity and scientific directness.

"The power of vitamin E to treat and prevent heart disease of all types, whether coronary or rheumatic, depends upon four chief characteristics:

(1) "Vitamin E seems to be a natural antithrombin in the human bloodstream. It has been found by Zierler of Johns Hopkins and the U. S. Navy Research Department and Kay at Tulane to be a substance normally circulating in the blood of all men, which prevents clotting occurring inside the vessel. It is the only substance preventing the clotting which is not dangerous. It does not interfere with the normal clotting of blood in a wound and with the normal healing process. Indeed, it actually accelerates the healing of burns and wounds.

(2) "The second important effect of the use of

the vitamin E is oxygen conservation. It is a natural antioxidant in the body. It has been shown by Houchin and Mattill, and this had been confirmed by many workers, to decrease the oxygen requirement of muscle by as much as 43 percent and makes the narrow stream of blood which gets through the narrowed coronary artery in many heart patients adequate to prevent the occurrence of anoxia (lack of oxygen), which is the trigger that sets off anginal or heart pain. Consequently, we have patients in Montreal who were once unable to walk half a block without the occurrence of angina pectoris but are now able to climb Mount Royal. Indeed, there is present in my audience today at least one such patient.

(3) "The third major function of vitamin E is the prevention of excessive scar tissue production and even, in some instances, the ability to melt away unwanted scar. It has been made known to us by given proof of its function this way in many areas of the body—from the hand, in Dupuytren's contraction (Rochester, N. Y.) to urinary tract strictures (Johns Hopkins).

(4) "It is a dilator of blood vessels. This was beautifully demonstrated by x-ray in rabbits injected before and after the administration of vitamin E by two workers in Florence, Italy. It opens up new pathways in the damaged circulation, therefore, and by-passes blocks produced by clots and hardened arteries.

"These four functions, all of them extensively

confirmed in animal experimentation and human clinical work, make it the most valuable ally the cardiologist has yet found in the treatment of heart disease. It has no rivals. No other substance has this array of needful properties. This drug then becomes the first safe drug which can be given to patients suffering from the results of clot in a coronary artery. There has been and still is no treatment at all for this type of case except two mildly useful drugs, which can be administered with great peril to the already precarious patient. Vitamin E replaces 'rest and reassurance,' (which have no authentic bases) with real help to the damaged, laboring heart. It is the key both to the prevention and treatment of all those conditions in which a lack of blood supply due to thickened or blocked vessels or lack of oxygen is a major part of the whole story of the disease. As I have said, it has no rivals. No pharmacologist or internist can suggest another substance with all the powers and properties of this vitamin. *God made it unique and we ignore it at our peril.*"

CHAPTER XI

Prevention of Harmful Blood Clots

WHEN YOU cut your finger and the blood coagulates to form a scab, a marvelous mechanism is at work. With the help of the platelets, described earlier, your blood coagulates to form a solid barrier to keep the moving bloodstream within your body. People with hemophilia, whose blood lacks this vital ability to clot, can bleed to death from a minor injury.

Within the vessels themselves, however, the blood should not clot, and when it does you are in for trouble. A blood clot within an artery can cut off the flow of blood and therefore the oxygen to any part of the body where it happens to get jammed. A clot in the arteries leading to the brain causes one major type of "stroke." If a clot becomes lodged in the coronary arteries, you have a "heart attack." Blockage of a major artery, in either of these two cases, usually means death.

As we noted earlier, clots form in the veins as well as the arteries. Indeed, they are particularly apt to form in the veins of the legs, for here the blood tends to be sluggish, having to fight against gravity in the long pull uphill to the abdomen and back to the heart. Thrombophlebitis—an inflamed vein in which a blood clot has developed—is a common disorder of the legs in older persons. If the clot breaks off and is carried in the bloodstream, its most dangerous destination is the lungs, for it probably will be carried safely through the large chambers and valves of the heart, but, if it gets to the lungs (a pulmonary embolism), it can cause grave damage.

It seems clear that something has gone wrong with body mechanisms when a lifesaving phenomenon—blood clotting—becomes a major factor in cardiovascular disease and death. One wonders: what are the natural regulators—those that nature provides to prevent coagulation within the vessels while keeping the mechanism always alert to stem external bleeding? If you will recall what Dr. Wilfrid Shute had to say about vitamin E at the close of the last chapter, you will suspect that this vitamin is one of the important regulators that nature intended us to have. He stated:

"Vitamin E seems to be a natural anti-thrombin in the human bloodstream. It has been found by Zierler of Johns Hopkins and the U. S. Navy Research Department and Kay at Tulane to be a substance normally circulating in the blood of all men, which prevents clotting occurring inside the vessel. It is the only substance preventing the clotting which is not dangerous. It does not interfere with the normal clotting of blood in a wound and with the normal healing process. Indeed, it actually accelerates the healing of burns and wounds."

It was in 1958, at the World Congress of Obstetrics and Gynecology in Montreal, that the Doctors Shute first presented their pioneering research on vitamin E. At that time they said, in connection with blood clotting:

"For example it (vitamin E) decreases embolism (blood clots) to the merest minimum. It not only prevents extension of existing clots, as do the classical anticoagulants, but it quickly resolves what clot is present. It acts very rapidly, especially in relieving associated pain and tenderness. It has none of the side effects which dog the anticoagulants, since it never produces hemorrhage, for example. Moreover, it does not require frequent blood examinations, can be self-administered far from any hospital or even medical care, and is as useful for clots in the vital organs as for clots in the peripheral vessels."

In diseases involving blood clots it has been customary to give certain drugs which keep the blood from coagulating. This seems like a good idea except for one thing—when you are destroying those substances in the blood that make it clot, how are you going to know when to stop? Carrying the treatment too far will bring about a condition where the thickening power of the blood is seriously disturbed and then hemorrhages are likely to follow.

A blood clot is indeed a serious thing, especially if it occurs in a blood vessel leading to the brain or the heart. Permanent damage or death may result. But a hemorrhage into either of these organs can be just as serious. When you begin to tamper with the blood's ability to clot, you can see that you can get into serious trouble. Vitamin E does not work this way. It is a natural constituent of the body—not a drug. So, instead, it regulates those substances in the blood that cause clotting or hemorrhaging.

Since vitamin E is so largely removed in modern food processing, a sensible preventive measure against internal blood clotting would be eating foods high in this vitamin, such as wheat germ, and supplementary vitamin E.

Another natural and safe block to clotting within the blood vessels may be onions. A Burma-born heart researcher at the Royal Victoria Infirmary in Newcastle upon Tyne, England, recently presented findings to this effect in the *British Medical Journal.* As reported in *Time* magazine (March 28, 1969), Dr. I. Sudhakaran Menon had heard that, in some parts of the world, a horse that develops clots in his legs is treated with a diet of garlic and onions. The researcher decided to test the onion theory on humans and enlisted the help of 22 volunteer patients at the Royal Victoria.

Dr. Menon fed his patients breakfasts high in fat, since a fat-loaded meal weakens the anti-clotting factors in the blood sharply within two or three hours. On one day the patients received 3 1/4 ounces of fat in their breakfasts, but no onions; on the next day, the same breakfast was served with 2 ounces of onions added. Without onions, the patients' blood-borne protections against clotting promptly dropped. With onions—whether served fried or boiled—their levels of anti-clotting factors rose rather than fell.

Just what it is in onions that offers this protection Dr. Menon says he does not know but he intends to investigate further.

An interesting theory about blood clotting was suggested some years ago by Dr. Ernest Klein, a New York physician, who found evidence during World War II that a high count of hemoglobin (the red coloring matter in blood) and a shortened coagulation period seemed to be typical of coronary thrombosis patients—patients who had suffered from clots in the coronary arteries. He argued from this observation that, if these two factors—coagulation time and hemoglobin count—could be kept normal, the danger of clotting inside the blood vessels would be lessened.

Later, at the Post-Graduate (now University) Hospital in New York, he checked his observations further in the hospital's blood donor center. Here he was put in charge of testing the hemoglobin, the condition of the heart and so forth, of all donors. For three years he had the opportunity of examining the blood of perhaps several hundred people a day. And he had the chance to get their cooperation in testing out various diets to find which diet would reduce a high hemoglobin count and lengthen a short coagulation time. At the end of a few days or weeks he could once again test their blood and determine whether or not the diet had accomplished what he wanted.

Drawing from this experience, Dr. Klein recommended—for those with high hemoglobin count—a plentiful intake of a mixture of fruit juice and water to thin the blood and a diet restricted in dry foods, such as bread, potatoes, cake, etc. A brief report on Dr. Klein's work appeared (May 20, 1949) in *New York Medicine*.

In recent years it has become necessary to warn against a new factor in the causation of blood clots: oral contraceptives. What once was considered primarily a disease of the older population now is a threat to young women of child-bearing age—thanks to "the pill" and the reckless way it has been promoted with scant regard to its side effects.

Although evidence has been building up at least since 1964, it was not until May, 1968 that the Food and Drug Administration finally got around to new labeling requirements warning of the pills' hazards. At that time, the FDA sent warning letters to the nation's 309,000 physicians. The agency cited findings recently published by British researchers that those who take the pill increase their chances of death or disease due to blood clots by seven to ten times. (*New York Times,* May 11, 1968.) The British studies showed the highest risks of thromboembolic deaths and diseases in women between the ages of 35 and 44.

A warning label, for the benefit of physicians and druggists, is now required on all shipments of oral contraceptives. Advertisements also must reflect the revised labeling. The label must state that a statistically significant association has been demonstrated between the use of oral contraceptives and thrombophlebitis and pulmonary embolism.

Clearly it is wooing disease to take these pills. The sooner American women make up their minds to give up this daily drug, the better for all concerned.

Finally, for all people, young and old, male and female, a specific preventive measure against blood clots is regular sustained exercise. Exercise, indeed, is essential to all aspects of cardiovascular health and will be discussed at greater length in Part III.

CHAPTER XII

Weight Gain and Loss

Doctors are fond of saying that you can add more years to your life—as well as more life to your years—by maintaining your body weight at the level best for you. Additional dividends of controlling your weight will be specific benefits to your blood pressure and circulatory system.

Why, you may ask, does reducing just a little make much difference to the body's plumbing system? Some basic facts will make this clear.

A pound of flesh contains from 30 to 50 feet of blood vessels, and your heart must keep these tubes supplied every minute of the day and night. Your heart was designed to do this, naturally, and it will do it very well—provided that you stay at the weight that your specific heart was designed to handle. Here, of course, is the rub—we don't *stay* at the optimal weight nature decrees, which in normal cases is the weight we arrive at about the time we're 20 years old. Our slowing up in the exercise department means that we stop burning up our food intake as fast as usual. And obviously, if we stop burning the fire so bright but continue to add the usual amount of fuel (or increase it, as we do all too often as we grow older), we are bound to start storing this unused fuel in the form of fat.

Many people rationalize that glandular imbalances are what makes them fat. Such disorders, however, are few and far between. The main cause of overweight, pure and simple, is too much food.

And too much food usually means too much of the *wrong* food. It's very seldom that you become overweight on a balanced diet. You never heard a doctor say, "You're fat because you eat too much protein and minerals." It's sugar and starch and other harmful carbohydrates that put on the weight.

There are many types of diets available for those who wish to lose or gain weight. The low-calorie diets that have become so popular should be viewed with suspicion, however, because they are frequently processed foods, artificially sweetened. Some of them are adequate to the job they say they do, but they should be examined carefully before use—and never indulged in to excess.

Far more satisfactory is a diet of natural foods that provide all the vital food elements that nature intends you to have, without making you fat. There is a certain amount of experimenting that one must indulge in to determine the best diet for one's individual needs; but one should continue trying and learning. Nothing can be of more permanent value than a balanced diet of natural foods that leaves one satisfied after each meal.

First, there is the question of how much and what kind of starchy food should be in the diet. In referring to starchy foods one often throws potatoes, bananas and bread in the same category as if the three of them act alike. But that is far from the case. Potatoes and bananas are nowhere near as fattening as bread, cake, cereals and other wheat products.

When you cut out bread you are also eliminating the salt that is in it, which is a factor in weight reducing. Dr. A. B. Anderson, writing in *The Lancet* of August 1, 1953 says, "In 1944 in a study of the weight loss of obese patients on submaintenance diets, I found that the greater weight loss of obese subjects on high-fat diets, as compared with those on high-carbohydrate diets, of equal caloric value, was due to the higher salt content of the high-carbohydrate diet, leading to retention of water and salt. When the salt content of the high-carbohydrate diet was reduced to that of the high-fat diet, the loss of weight was the same on both diets. It is often found that after putting the patient on such a diet there is very little loss of weight at first, owing to water retention, and the patient is disappointed and loses faith in the treatment. If a low-salt diet is given from the beginning, the weight loss begins at once, to the satisfaction of both patient and practitioner."

Dr. Anderson, of course, in mentioning salt-containing carbohydrates is referring mainly to bread and cereals made of wheat.

In its November 1956 issue, *Esquire* described a method of losing up to 30 pounds in 60 days with its *Deamof* diet. *Deamof* stands for "Don't eat anything made of flour." This means no bread, toast, buns, biscuits, corn bread, cookies, cakes, gravies, sauces, pancakes, puddings, pies, popovers, breakfast foods, spaghetti, ravioli, noodles, etc. Eat anything else says this article and you'll still lose the 30 pounds in 60 days. According to the article, quite a few persons tried the diet and found that it worked.

Incidentally, it is not only the salt in the bread that causes the increase in the weight. There is something more, probably the gluten, which makes the bread rise in the baking. That is why other forms of starch that contain no gluten, such as potatoes and bananas, are not nearly as fattening. Also bear in mind that wheat contains 2 1/2 percent fat, bananas only 1/2 of 1 percent, white potatoes 1/10 of 1 percent and sweet potatoes 1.1 percent fat.

There are many things wrong with wheat. It causes celiac disease in children, and this condition is increasing alarmingly. An overconsumption of bread and cereals by children, due to the phytate content of the wheat, robs calcium from the bones and causes rickets. The chemical chlorides added to the flour for various purposes destroy vitamin E in the human body—that vitamin so necessary to cardiac health. Wheat is very acid and plays a large part in producing the condition of acidosis which lowers the resistance of the body to bacterial infection. Writing in the *American Journal of Digestive Diseases and Nutrition*, September, 1937, Drs. Irwin Spiesman and Lloyd Arnold of the Illinois College of Medicine reported that colds were reduced greatly in patients with chronic colds by eliminating all wheat products from their diet. There is also evidence that eye diseases associated with catarrhal conditions may be rapidly benefited by the restriction of bread carbohydrates.

If you are a heart case you owe it to yourself to eliminate all wheat products and see what happens. This means complete elimination—not even a slice of toast a day, and absolutely no sandwiches of any kind.

Now you will say, if I can't eat bread, what shall I substitute? Fruit and potatoes. Since breakfast is the one meal where the average person will miss his toast and breakfast food, here is a typical wheatless breakfast: two fairly good-sized sweet potatoes; two hard-boiled eggs; eight stewed prunes; a serving of applesauce (homemade without added sugar) covered with wheat germ flakes; rose hip tea.

This fills you up so thoroughly that you can wait four or five hours before eating lunch. Sweet potatoes are an ideal starch food, very rich in vitamin A, very tasty and nonfattening. White potatoes are very healthful too. A whole book could be written on the potato and its health-giving qualities. It has been almost the sole food of whole races of people. It is practically self-contained—rich in vitamins and minerals, and its effect is alkaline on the body if consumed with the skin. We cannot say that of wheat.

The breakfast outlined above weighs about a pound and a half, sometimes two pounds, but it is nonfattening because it has all day long to work itself off. Our recommended lunch weighs about one pound and so does the evening meal. They are uniform meals consisting of a small portion of lean meat, vegetables, including raw peas, some sunflower seeds, and rose hip tea. A few hours after supper, eat some raw fruit. On this diet you will lose weight consistently.

The heart case should consume a low-fat diet. Then why eat two eggs a day? The answer is that, on this diet, eggs are practically the sole source of fat. You eat no fried foods, no milk, butter, cheese, cream or ice cream, and the meats are those that contain less fat such as chicken and turkey. Steaks and other beef cuts are high on the fat meat list.

It is important to reduce the total amount of fat in the diet of a person with a heart condition, but in making the decision as to which types of fat to retain in the diet, bear in mind that the egg is a whole food, out of which a living thing will emerge. It has the germ of life in it if it is a fertile egg. There just isn't any comparison with milk and dairy products. The egg is by far superior from every point of view, besides containing a large quantity of lecithin which is the antidote to the cholesterol that the egg contains. To cut down on eggs is a terrible dietary blunder even where there is hardening of the arteries.

Skipping breakfast as a means of losing weight is not desirable. That is the opinion of many medical experts. The consensus is that you will be so hungry that you will eat more the rest of the day. A heavy breakfast lulls your appetite the rest of the day. Thus, you will find it easy to eat very light lunches—one half the amount of food you used to eat.

A project at the State University of Iowa showed that breakfast skippers lose energy in the late morning hours and work with less efficiency. In Britain the Central Council for Health Education found that those who eat roast beef for breakfast have more energy, are more cheerful and will lose weight easily.

A proper protein breakfast including eggs and meat or fish automatically begins processes by which the body will use its own fat as an energy-giving fuel. But if breakfast is skipped, or if it is too light, these body processes will be frustrated, and too great demands will be made on the blood sugar. Such a person becomes irritable, weak and sickly.

Those who skip breakfasts tend to eat very large evening meals, which are dangerous for a heart case. In the morning when the fires of the body's metabolism are burning strongly, the body can easily burn up a big meal, so to speak. But this is not true in the evening when the processes of the body are at a lower ebb.

This is illustrated by the famous case of Alexander Parr, who in the times of Henry VIII lived to be about 150. His secret was extremely frugal eating. Henry VIII heard about Parr and invited him to come to the palace, where a huge banquet was given in his honor. Parr ate so much food that the next day he died.

Luigi Cornaro (1467-1565) is another illustration of how frugality in the diet causes a man to live long. Due to dissipations and intemperance in eating, Cornaro became very ill when he was about 40 and was given up by his physicians. He fooled them, however, by moving into the country where he worked out a bare subsistence diet, as a result of which he attained the age of 98. There is much medical evidence in experiments with rats proving conclusively that reduction in daily calories adds years to the life. But this is especially important to a heart case because the heart is overtaxed in helping to digest heavy meals.

Dr. Clive M. McCay of Cornell University found

that he could double the life span of rats by reducing their intake of food by one half. His rats which normally lived some 600 days, lived 1,068 days under the low food regimen. Professor Leonard A. Maynard commenting on this experiment said: "The eat-as-they-please rats had the shortest life-span; those that went on a diet in middle age lived longer. The oldest rat, which lived 1,400 days (equivalent to 140 years), never had a square meal in his life."

It all boils down to the fact that we live on about half of what we eat, and overtax our hearts by compelling them to work on the other half.

The following are to be eliminated from the diet if you wish to reduce, and to create the ideal conditions for the proper functioning of the heart:

fried foods	dairy products
coffee or tea or maté	sugar
soups	salt

bread and flour. etc.

This means no French fried potatoes (the 5th most popular food choice in the United States), and no soups. The average person on a reducing diet seems to be unaware of how fattening soups can be and how easy it is to get along without them. Soup is a liquid that pyschologically does not satisfy craving as much as foods that are solid. Also that fat content of soup is very dangerous for a heart case.

Of course one cannot cut out fats altogether. If one does, one may become the subject of feelings of depression. Fat is necessary for the proper absorption of carotene which is the first step in the body's manufacture of vitamin A. Egg yolk, which contains fat, is also very rich in iron, an element that many persons are deficient in. Incidentally, a hard-boiled egg will hold the hunger for a longer period than scrambled or medium-boiled eggs.

One must develop a little bag of tricks to fool the appetite, and also to study various processes of the body and the effect of food thereon. For example, salting food stimulates the appetite and makes one thirsty. This is important to know in the summer when people tend to consume soft drinks.

Cheese and such foods are appetite stimulators. These types of foods must be found out and if necessary eliminated from the diet. Some people claim that brewer's yeast increases their appetites. If that is the case, they should get their vitamin B from desiccated liver and wheat germ. An important thing is for the whole family to be on the same diet. Then no tempting foods like ice cream and cakes will be present to taunt one. If there were no ice cream in the world, it would soon be forgotten and it would not be missed. What a wonderful effect this would have on the health of everyone!

When one gets hungry after supper, there is nothing wrong in eating an apple or some lettuce or celery. These will add little if any weight. One of the fruits to guard against is the date, which has a high sugar content. Honey is good, but should be taken in moderation.

A method some people use to get off a few pounds, when they seem to be at rock bottom and it is difficult to make further progress, is to go to bed without any supper. They find that hunger goes away when they lie down. They usually take some interesting reading to bed. Although this is a difficult method, it is good for a loss of two to three pounds which would be otherwise very hard to slough off.

Another method that some find very effective is "the law of not even one," which means that, for example, if you have decided to cut out ice cream or cake, you never make an exception even if you are at a birthday party of a dear friend or at other celebrations. Once you begin to make one exception, your willpower becomes fuzzy, but if, on the other hand, you have made up your mind thoroughly, and never weaken, then your subconscious develops the habit of refusing, and refusals then come easy. It is a matter of educating your willpower.

Part Three: Guidelines for a Healthy Circulatory System

CHAPTER XIII

Exercise Puts Real Life Into Your Arteries

EXERCISE IS OF tremendous importance to the blood pressure and circulatory system. This accounts for the link between heart fatalities and sedentary workers which has been confirmed in a remarkable study of 191,609 railroad men made by University of Minnesota researchers.

The researchers asked, "Do active jobs offer some protection against heart disease?" and then used electric computers to analyze Railroad Retirement Board records of men from 40 to 64 years old with at least ten years' railroad service.

Office workers were considered sedentary workers. Switchmen were classed as those who engage in a moderate amount of physical activity. Section men comprised the heavy labor group. The results were startling, showing that the death rate from heart disease was 5.7 per thousand office workers in all age groups—more than twice the 2.8 rate for section men! The death rate for switchmen was 3.9.

Many other studies of this type have by now firmly established the relationship of physical activity to the development of coronary artery disease.

About ten years ago British researchers compared bus drivers with conductors, and mail carriers with office workers. They found that the conductors who climbed up and down London's double-decker buses all day long to collect fares had fewer deaths from cardiac ailments than the more sedentary bus drivers. Heart deaths for postmen also were lower than those of office workers.

Elsewhere on the research front, scientists are checking on such factors as heredity, environment, diet, and vitamin supplements in the never-ending study of heart and circulatory ills.

Dr. J. R. Winston, medical director of the Santa Fe Railroad, stated in that road's magazine: "During the past 20 years we have witnessed more spectacular developments in the control of heart disease than our forebears observed in the previous 300 years." He added that the greatest potential for advancement in heart research lies in the area of prevention—"prevention of all types of heart and blood vessel diseases."

Who is the potential cardiac case? Dr. Paul Dudley White says a man with a family history of cardiac disease is more likely to become a heart victim himself than if he has no such background. And, the famed heart expert points out, so is a fellow with a hard-driving ambition, a penchant for fat-rich foods and heavy smoking, and a disregard for regular physical exercise.

Dr. White attended the late Dwight D. Eisenhower, when the then president was stricken by heart disease. It was Dr. White who was responsible for getting Eisenhower to cut out cigarettes and take time from his White House duties for more outdoor exercise on the golf links.

Dr. White, of course, practices what he preaches. In his late 70's, he climbs mountains, splits wood, jogs, and rides a bicycle. The benefits of such exercise are summed up by Dr. Hans Selye, noted Canadian scientist, who says, "By exercising intelligently, a man can train his heart to resist attacks that otherwise might kill him." Dr. Selye, you will recall, also puts great emphasis on the relationship between heart disease and vitamins and trace minerals. Exercise he sees as part of the total program of prevention.

Many a person with a heart condition who suffers angina or chest pains when beginning a walk, will soon discover that in many cases these disappear if the walk is continued for more than 15 minutes. The exercise oxygenates and dilates the arteries. At the beginning of the walk the heart, suddenly being asked to go into action, finds that it doesn't have enough oxygen to keep it working at the increased rate demanded. But the deficit is soon wiped out by the effect of the continued exercise.

An inactive person who is a heart case and who suddenly is forced to move fast will find himself in trouble. But if his heart has become used to exercise, it will readjust itself more easily to emergency demands. We might safely state that lack of exercise is one of the causes of heart disease. It is thoroughly proven in medical literature. Today there is no question about this. But let us see what lack of exercise does to some of the other organs of the body.

In the *American Practitioner and Digest of Treatment* (July, 1956), appears the following: "Towbin has shown that the incidence of pulmonary embolism (the blocking of an artery in the lungs) is probably much higher than generally supposed. Many aged persons who supposedly die from cardiac disease probably die as the result of pulmonary embolism. Thrombophlebitis (a condition in which inflammation of the vein wall has preceded the formation of the clot in the vein) of the legs with its resultant pulmonary embolism is caused to some extent by lack of exercise."

Dr. Otto Meyer, of New York, who specialized in phlebitis, effected miraculous cures by injections and bandaging of the feet of the patient and then advising him to walk a great deal every day. Dr. Meyer's patients were usually people who stood a great deal but did not move around much, such as dentists, floorwalkers, barbers, etc. He claimed that it was lack of movement that was at the bottom of phlebitis.

The Lancet (July 2, 1966) reported on a group of eight male and one female middle-aged patients with coronary disease, who were examined before and after a month of training on a bicycle. Training sessions lasted 30 minutes, and the work load for each person was increased by 50 percent every five minutes. Patients pedaled at the laboratory every day during the first week, and every other day during the following week. Doctors found that the work load tolerated by the patients could be increased considerably toward the end of the training period. In fact, the working-capacity increased in all patients.

The patients agreed that a strikingly heavier degree of exertion was necessary to cause any chest pain or breathlessness after training than before. Blood pressure was slightly but not significantly lower after training. Hemoglobin values rose slightly and consistently after the training, and the hemoglobin capacity of the blood increased in all the patients but one. Doctors concluded that all patients improved clinically and had increased exercise tolerance with respect to angina pectoris and dizziness.

Nutrition Reviews (July, 1967) printed new evidence that serum cholesterol levels may be kept significantly lower by means of regularly performed endurance exercises. Among the recent studies that confirm the effect of physical conditioning in this field is the work of S. R. Shane who evaluated 877 flying personnel at the School of Aerospace Medicine from 1963-1964. They had all undergone treadmill exercise testing and had their cholesterol levels determined. The results showed that both serum cholesterol and triglyceride levels showed a significant down-trend after a workout on the treadmill.

A very interesting finding about an athlete's heart is discussed in *The New England Journal of Medicine,* November, 1961. Dr. James H. Currens at autopsy examined the heart of Clarence de Mar, known to sports fans as Mr. Marathon, who died of cancer at the age of 70 in April, 1958. He discovered that Mr. de Mar's heart was fed by a coronary artery two or three times the normal diameter and stated that this was due, no doubt, to the great amount of physical exercise that had made demands upon the arteries.

It is also known that in athletes the heart becomes enlarged and the pulse beat slower, all through exercise. Many physicians have stated that intense athletics weaken the heart. This now seems completely disproven by the studies of many medical research workers.

It is amazing what the body can do to adjust itself to unusual situations. For example, it has been found that, when a person exercises a great deal, new capillaries are made by the body to take care of the additional needs of the new activity. But that the blood vessels can enlarge themselves through exercise is a startling new finding.

The hesitation that grips most recovering cardiac patients when it comes to exercise is perfectly understandable. They're afraid they might overdo it and have another attack. Many doctors still hesitate to prescribe exercise for the same reasons. Others act as though the sky's the limit, and a patient can do anything. In the *British Medical Journal* (March 9, 1968) Drs. J. Schouten and J. Schreuder suggest: "If the physician will take the time to walk with his patients a few times he generally does not need elaborate methods to make an adequate training program. He can use his simple objective observations as a measure of the patient's tolerance to exercise."

The authors disagree strongly with the general tendency to find the maximum effort of which a patient is capable after recovering from myocardial infarction—for example, pedaling on a bicycle to see how well he can hold out before exhaustion. "This way of thinking seems to us unphysiological and dangerous. On the contrary, no patient should exercise at maximum speed, not even experimentally and under electrocardiographic control. . . . Our method is to begin with exercise in bed, and when the patient is mobilized we take him walking. Initial speed, the period of adaptation, the maximum speed is thus determined."

Most doctors agree that every organ in the body is benefited by exercise of its function. This includes the heart. The question is how much exercise is beneficial before it starts to be dangerous? Surely in a life or death situation, most doctors would be willing to take a short walk with the patient, just to be on the safe side in prescribing exercise.

CHAPTER XIV

Dangers of Many Drugs

Digitalis, the old war horse and standby among cardiac medications, had its pedestal shaken by Dr. Albert N. Brest, director of the Cardiovascular Research Institute at Hahnemann Hospital. Speaking at the Pennsylvania Medical Society's annual meeting, October, 1967, he cautioned that digitalis can "do considerable harm" under certain conditions. Toxic reactions to digitalis are "too commonly" encountered, said Brest, largely because it is used in some cases of heart failure where it really has no application. Dr. Brest added this: "There is evidence from animal experiments that with decreased serum magnesium there is increased sensitivity to digitalis toxicity. This occurs even with normal potassium levels." Presumably, the problems with digitalis are less likely to occur in patients using a magnesium supplement such as dolomite.

The main danger involved here is that most doctors think of digitalis as a completely harmless drug, and once they have prescribed its use they relax and let the patient go on using it indefinitely on a maintenance dose. Dr. Arnold S. Moe, writing in the Illinois Medical Journal (June, 1959), told of 100 cases of digitalis poisoning, originally reported in the *Texas Medical Journal* (October. 1956). It was found that .2 milligrams of digitalis, taken as a daily maintenance dose, proved to be toxic. Twenty-seven of the hundred patients died (presumably from their heart ailments) and seven of these deaths were directly attributed to digitalis. The heart patient who is receiving digitalis must be watched carefully. In the *Journal of the American Medical Association* (April 26, 1958) an article touching on the subject, by L. Craig and his colleagues, contained this statement: "Average dose formulas, as well as other dogmatic over-simplifications in prescriptions of digitalis drugs, disregard biologic variability. In other words, it is not likely that the same continued dosage will be beneficial for a man weighing 200 pounds, and for a woman weighing 98 pounds, even though their blood pressure readings might be similar. One is bound to be getting too small a dose, or the other too much. Great discretion and careful observation for effects should characterize all digitalis prescriptions."

An illustration of how the use of digitalis can get

out of hand is offered in Dr. Moe's case history of a 60-year-old male patient who came to a physician's office complaining that he had suffered a "heart spell," characterized by rapid beating of the heart. Digitalis was prescribed at first, and later the man was put on a maintenance dose of one and one half tablets of digitalis per day. He was under instructions to increase the maintenance dose by one tablet if the heart should begin beating rapidly again. About a month later he noticed that he had begun to speak nothing but nonsense, sometimes for a day or two at a time, but he could not control what he was saying. His eyes became irritated and were playing color tricks on him. Visits to several eye specialists showed no physiological disturbances of the eyes.

The patient began to suspect that the digitalis was the cause of his new difficulties, but his doctor seriously warned him against lowering or discontinuing his digitalis dosage. The patient had a thorough physical examination, and there was no abnormality of any organ. Even the heart did not show any serious defect. Digitalis was discontinued. In six days the patient felt his color vision was improving and in six weeks he felt it was back to normal. The pulse rate also returned to a normal range as did the blood pressure. It was concluded by the last physician he saw that the patient's "heart spell" was nothing more than palpitations, a common heart-pounding sensation which is not always an indication of heart disease.

In *Medical Press* (December 16, 1959), Dr. Frank W. Law, surgeon at Morfield's Eye Hospital in London, wrote that digitalis threatens the user with an unique side effect on the eyes. Vision may become monochrome, everything in one color—red, yellow or green. Digitalis was cited as a cause of visual hallucinations.

The problem is that many of the other time-honored drugs are not much better, and in many instances are worse than digitalis, in terms of safety and reliability.

Quinidine is another popular drug used in treating circulatory disorders, especially where irregular heartbeat is a factor. It is often employed in an attempt to prevent heart failure. Dr. Moe tells us that a single small dose of this drug, improperly administered, might be fatal. More commonly the toxic effects of quinidine are: nausea, vomiting, epigastric distress, headache, diarrhea, apprehension and ringing in the ears. Sometimes visual disturbances, fever, and skin rashes result from its use.

In *Circulation* (November, 1956), G. W. Thompson reported on 611 cases collected from literature, and, of these, death in 2.1 percent was attributed to quinidine. Quinidine is known as a classic drug for treating excessively rapid heartbeat. A case history of a 53-year-old male heart patient shows the danger of depending exclusively on such a drug. The man experienced episodes of rapid heartbeat for five years. He was admitted to the hospital when one such episode lasted much longer than usual. Quinidine, the classic drug in such cases, was prescribed in increasing doses. It almost killed the patient. His pulse rate went from 146 to 240 per minute. Digitalis was employed as an alternate just in time, and the patient recovered.

Hexamethosium was widely used, at first, to lower blood pressure. It works, but the toxic effects that can accompany it have cut into its popularity: constipation, blurring vision, bowel obstruction, prostatic obstruction, and a sudden and extreme drop in blood pressure when a patient with advanced hardening of the arteries rises to a standing position.

Hydralazine is used for hypertension. When it is, dizziness, rapid heartbeat and headache are likely to follow. But most alarming, hydralazine has been known to *produce* angina pectoris in some patients.

Nitroglycerin, a drug used for heart trouble, may give temporary beneficial effects, according to the *Medical Journal of Australia* for November 5, 1955, but it may also overbalance these good effects and go too far in the other direction, resulting in circulatory collapse and fainting.

Rauwolfia, the father of the tranquilizers, is used extensively in one form or another for relief of hypertension. The *Journal of the American Medical Association* (September 8, 1956) reported on 56 cases treated with rauwolfia. Four of these developed severe anxiety, agitation and depression. As for the other side effects, 82 percent of the 56 patients developed drowsiness, fatigue, weight loss, loss of initiative and nightmares.

Another example of the undesirability of rauwolfia was cited in the *American Journal of Medical Science* (August, 1956). Investigators Bello and Turner showed, by means of a double-blind test, that reserpine (a rauwolfia drug) caused neither consistent nor adequate blood pressure reduction. Two-thirds of the cases used in the test showed the common rauwolfia side effects.

So these are the drugs used by most physicians in treating heart disorders. True, there are times when their effectiveness cannot be denied. but it would be difficult, in the face of the evidence provided by Dr. Moe, to insist on their absolute safety. Further to refuse to use vitamin E, due to concern over its side effects, and then to use any of the drugs mentioned above instead, is hardly consistent.

Not only drugs used specifically for cardiac disorders but other drugs too can damage the heart. Harmful side effects from estrogen therapy have been making the medical journals for more than a generation. Recently Veterans Administration studies showed that victims of prostate cancer who are treated with hormones die quicker with the therapy than without it. Now, perhaps we know why. According to Dr. John C. Bailer III, "Estrogen therapy may increase the risk of early death in all but the most advanced cases of prostatic cancer . . . you will not realize the dangers of hormone treatment unless you study the cardiovascular problems common to the age group."

Dr. Bailer's Veterans Administration study of 2,300 patients indicates that prostate victims without hormone and castration treatment have fewer heart attacks or strokes than those who have estrogen doses. According to *Science News* (August 19, 1967), Dr. Bailer warns that physicians "should carefully weigh the benefits of hormone treatment against the hazards."

Doctors are puzzled by occasional fatalities in which the victims simply keel over with no sign of struggle or distress, and nothing more shows up in postmortems. Doctors at Veterans Administration Hospital, North Little Rock, Arkansas, and the University of Arkansas Medical Center believe they have come up with the answer: the long, heavy use of various tranquilizers might be a cause of heart damage.

Writing in the *Journal of the American Medical Association* (January 24, 1966), the Arkansas researchers—Drs. Howard L. Richardson, Kathryn I. Graupner and Mary E. Richardson—reported on their investigation of deaths from unknown causes. Microscopic studies of the hearts of four men—all long-time tranquilizer users—who had died suddenly, revealed degeneration of the inner heart muscle tissue and blood vessels. The defects apparently threw off the heart's rhythmic balance, the researchers noted. Similar defects were produced in the hearts of animals fed phenothiazine tranquilizers and subjected to conditions of stress, they explained.

In summary, drugs are never preferable to nutritional remedies where there is a genuine choice between the two. As scientific evidence continues to mount on the effectiveness of vitamin and mineral therapy and proper diet, we believe these measures will emerge as the best of all treatments for cardiac diseases.

CHAPTER XV

Other Harmful Substances

CERTAIN TRACE METALS are essential for the body's welfare, as we have seen in Chapter nine. Other metals, however, can be harmful. Dr. Henry A. Schroeder, whose work on beneficial metals we reported earlier, believes that there are abnormal metals present in the tissues of modern Americans and that these may be a cause of hardening of the arteries. He reported his findings in *The Journal of Chronic Diseases,* July, 1955.

The traces of these harmful substances are apparently deposited in the body when people are exposed to them over a period of time during their everyday activities.

For instance, an examination of human tissues may reveal little or no cobalt (which is absolutely essential for health) but relatively large amounts of nickel and chromium. Where could the nickel come from? One very likely source is the process of hydrogenation. When healthful vegetable oils like corn oil, peanut oil, cottonseed oil and so forth, are made solid by hydrogenation, much of that precious unsaturated fatty acid is destroyed. In addition, as Dr. Schroeder says, "It is interesting that nickel catalysts are used in the hydrogenation of edible vegetable oils."

Could this be one of the main reasons why, in a table Dr. Schroeder gives showing the minerals present in human tissues, there should be, in general, such large concentrations of nickel, especially compared to the amounts of essential minerals like manganese and cobalt?

Why should human tissues in our century also show such large concentrations of aluminum unless it is because of the widespread use of aluminum cooking utensils, foil wrappings on food and other sources of contamination by aluminum to which much of our food has been exposed? Is it not possible that concentrations of these metals that are not essential to human beings may displace the mineral that is supposed to act along with certain members of the B vitamin complex in metabolizing fat in the human body, asks Dr. Schroeder.

A reader queried the *Journal of the American Medical Association* (December 10, 1960) as follows: "In a current study of the metal content of aging aortic tissue it was noted . . . that the metal that contributes to aging change is probably not calcium but rather aluminum, manganese or copper. What is the biochemistry and enzymatic chemistry involved in this aging process? From what sources would the aluminum probably come?"

The authority assigned by the *Journal* to answer the question states that it is difficult to determine just how much any given tissue contains of trace minerals. But he believes that trace minerals which are not easily assimilated would tend to accumulate in the body. He says that little is known about the function of aluminum in the body. "It is undoubtedly poorly absorbed," he goes on, "but estimates of 100 micrograms have been made for the average amount absorbed per day. . . . Certain plants accumulate aluminum salts and these salts are present in small concentrations in drinking water, usually much less than 1 part per million."

The article referred to by the *Journal* questioner above—"The Metal Content Correlation in Aging Aorta," by H. H. Zinsser and two associates at the University of Southern California Medical School—appeared in the *Journal of the American Geriatrics Society,* January, 1957. The authors state that there seems to be abundant evidence that the aorta becomes increasingly less elastic with age. Using an electron microscope these researchers found, they say, that the accumulation of minerals did not appear to be calcium. They found that, for all metals except manganese, there was a definite increase with age. For calcium, copper, iron and lead there were fairly large increases with age. Deposits of aluminum were significantly increased in all the samples.

Discussing the quite large amounts of aluminum that they found, the investigators go on to remark that aluminum is used commercially in certain combinations of chemicals *specifically for the purpose of giving rigidity*. Thus it seems that it may be responsible for just such a result in the human blood vessel.

The authors say that they have subjected only a few blood vessels to the exhaustive, exacting trial tests they outline. They state that more researchers should take up the question of the accumulation of metals in the arteries. But they also state: "There are good reasons for minimizing the key role that calcium has been given in the development of the elastic changes in the aging aorta. . . . Aluminum would account most satisfactorily for the multiple bonding and increases in rigidity. . . . Manganese and copper remain possible agents."

It is quite possible that aluminum is too active a metal to be used for the many things we use it for today, in relation to food. Aluminum cooking utensils are particularly suspect because when foods, especially acid foods, are heated in such utensils, they take up aluminum from the pans. There seems to be no doubt that this is so, but we have always been told by "the authorities" and the Better Business Bureau that such contamination of food by aluminum could not possibly be harmful. The canning industry has gone ahead with manufacture of food cans of aluminum rather than tin. Aluminum foil is used to wrap many of the things we buy, in addition to being very inexpensively available for home use.

If indeed aluminum is not easily absorbed by the body, if it accumulates in arteries, as the studies above seem to indicate, then by escaping as much aluminum exposure as we can, we may be able to postpone longer that gradual process of hardening which creates such difficulty for our heart and circulatory system. Perhaps aluminum is only a small part of one aspect of this problem. Perhaps the widespread home use of copper water pipes with its slight contamination of drinking water with copper contributes its part, as well. And undoubtedly other metals which are ingested in water and food contribute to the whole picture.

But if we can avoid even a small part of this dismal accumulation in the linings of arteries, we will be doing ourselves a favor. If, in addition to avoiding contamination by metals we also follow the best possible diet, getting plenty of the B vitamins and the right kind of fats and shunning refined carbohydrates and processed fats, perhaps we can avoid the almost inevitable hardening of the arteries altogether.

In making decisions as to whether to buy things made of metal, the criterion to apply to aluminum and other metals is: do they actually contaminate things that I eat or drink? Obviously an aluminum chair or roof or a copper bottom on the outside of a kettle do not contaminate food or drink. So use these metals in any way you wish, *except in a way which might contaminate food or drink.*

Present-day inhabitants of Poland have less lead in their bones than the people of most other European countries and the United States. Researchers have had trouble explaining why Poles are so fortunate, but one chemist from the Warsaw Institute of Nuclear Research puts the difference down to western dietary habits and food contamination, according to *New Scientist* (January 18, 1968). He believes that high lead concentrations might once have been due to the use by Westerners of tin kitchen utensils, which contain a lot of lead. But today they use few tin utensils and high concentrations of lead still persist. These concentrations, says Dr. Jaworowski, must be due to some other feature in a way of life not present in Poland. It can't be the increasing industrial contamination, because Poland has that too. The logical variable, says Jaworowski, is what we eat, how we grow and process our foods. Pesticides, for one thing, contain enough lead to contaminate the crops they are intended to protect.

The French health magazine *La Vie Claire* recently warned of the harmful effects of cereals as follows:

"By this work on the mechanisms of assimilation of cereals, deLarebeyrette has succeeded in showing that certain cardiovascular diseases are diseases of assimilation. The origin of most cardiovascular troubles derives from defective function of the supra-renal glands whose normal secretions are indispensable to the assimilation of certain glucides. When the secretions of the supra-renal glands fail, the assimilation of the glucides deriving from cereals is weakened and the blood is filled with serum mucoids, which increase its viscosity and add to the circulatory insufficiency. This is how cardiovascular diseases are formed.

"But the process is metabolic in origin, exactly as in diabetes."

DeLarebeyrette is not the first researcher to incriminate wheat as a formidable barrier to a healthy heart. In 1958 Drs. John W. Gofman, Alex V. Nichols and E. Virginia Dobbin of the University of California, wrote a book, *Dietary Prevention and Treatment of Heart Disease,* published by G. P. Putnam, in which they spoke out against the effect of carbohydrates, in forming fatty deposits on the walls of the blood vessels.

Specifically they drew attention to the fact that some people were highly susceptible to a deleterious effect on the heart by eating wheat, but that the only way to tell was by a blood test. If you happen to be a wheat "susceptible," it could mean your life to stop eating wheat in every form.

Another physician, Dr. Robert R. Levin, M.D., spoke out against bread in the February, 1962 issue of *Connecticut Medicine,* as follows:

"Ofttimes I have achieved fabulous results with

cardiac or hypertensive patients by the simple expedient of forbidding the use of bread or flour products."

Another very common food in the American diet perhaps should be classified as a "harmful substance." According to *Science News,* November 5, 1966, Dr. Jackson Blair of Lakewood, Ohio, believes that table mustard is one of the causes of coronary disease, arteriosclerosis and high blood pressure. He also implicates pepper and ginger as possible causes of high blood pressure.

Dr. Blair reported on 12 cases of coronary disease where he found that the patients ate large amounts of mustard. There are certain chemicals in mustard, called esters, which he believes corrode the arteries.

Dr. Blair advises women especially against eating mustard, pepper and ginger, because in female rats they produced cysts in the ovaries, and it is very unusual for laboratory rats to get ovarian cysts. In the case of a woman these cysts often lead to surgery to remove the ovary. The doctor warns against products in which mustard is concealed such as mayonnaise and salad dressing.

Sufferers of circulatory disorders who may wonder whether or not drinking alcohol is beneficial will be interested in the findings of three U. S. Public Health Service researches that were published in the May 27, 1950, issue of the *Journal of the American Medical Association.* The authors found from electrocardiograms that alcohol does not open up the coronary (heart) arteries. They say that the prevailing idea that alcohol is good medicine for heart cases "should be drastically amended."

One of the researchers (Dr. Henry I. Russek) says that alcohol ingestion might actually be dangerous, even though an ounce or so of whiskey often stops the pain of angina. First, there is danger that the alcohol will remove the warning signal, which the pain is supposed to be. Dr. Russek says, "The view that a glass of whiskey is the equivalent of a glyceryl trinitrate tablet for the patient with coronary disease should be rejected."

Says *Science News Letter,* June 3, 1950, commenting on this research: "The whiskey, they found, did not prevent the changes in the electrocardiograms brought on by the exercise test, but the glyceryl trinitrate either completely prevented or significantly modified these changes. The whiskey did prevent the pain and other sensations of angina, however.

"Alcohol's effect in angina, they conclude, is due to its rapid action as a sedative. The tests with morphine bore this out. And while the sedative effect may be good for the patient having an attack of angina, it could be dangerous for a person to take whiskey before undertaking vigorous physical effort.

"The alcohol would not dilate his arteries, and would banish the danger signal of pain, thus perhaps putting him in the spot of undertaking more than his heart can stand. Sudden death or fatal seizure might be the result."

Another investigation shows that moderate or immoderate drinking of any kind of alcoholic beverages causes the red blood cells to stick to each other in clumps. This is dangerous because it slows down the speed of the blood flow, thus reducing the oxygen supply to the tissues. In heart disease it is important that there be a sufficient supply of oxygen going to the heart. This work was done in Finland by the State Alcohol Monopoly research laboratories and was reported in the *Quarterly Journal of Studies on Alcohol* (December, 1955).

It seems, therefore, that as far as heart cases are concerned, its best to be an absolute teetotaler.

Milk also should be listed among the foods to avoid. The word that milk brings on heart problems comes straight from the desk of noted authority Dr. Paul Dudley White. Heavy milk drinking among teen-agers, with other uses of animal fats beginning in childhood, might lead to the early development of clogged arteries or atherosclerosis, said Dr. White. He was speaking as a result of intensive investigation not only in the United States but in Japan, Italy and Greece.

CHAPTER XVI

Your Pulse and Your Heart

A WARNING of impending heart disease is usually signaled two to five years before the actual attack. This important fact was revealed in the *Medical Journal of Australia,* April 6, 1957, in an editorial which stated:

"A point of some importance in the early diagnosis of coronary disease, and in the detection of probable candidates for the disease in the future, is the observation that there is a sustained rise of pulse rate (15 to 30 beats per minute) and of diastolic pressure (10 to 30 millimetres of mercury) on the average of two to five years prior to attack." (The diastolic pressure is the one which is usually given second—for example, in 120 over 70, 70 is the diastolic pressure.)

In light of these findings, it would seem important—particularly for those over 50—to keep track of pulse rate as well as blood pressure. In earlier chapters we have dealt with blood pressure and various measures that can be taken to keep it within the normal range. The present chapter concerns the rate of the pulse. It is a personal account by J. I. Rodale, which appeared originally in the December, 1954 issue of *Prevention*.

A few months ago I completed the manuscript of a book called *This Pace is not Killing Me*. The main contention of the book is that not only are we *not* traveling at a faster pace, but that it is not the pace that kills. In fact, I showed that the reverse was true. Most heart cases die because of a killing inactivity. Their hearts cannot take such indolence.

When the book was completed I realized that I was the worst offender in regard to what I had written. I was the most typical example of the sedentary businessman that I had been so loudly censuring. Being 56, and a heart case, I can now see from what I have learned about the evils of inactivity that unless I change my way of life I am in for consequences. Only ten months ago I was turned down for life insurance. When I walk upgrade there comes a feeling of pressure in the chest region. It is difficult to pin down the exact nature of my condition. The doctors seem to be vague about it. One of them called it coronary sclerosis.

Have they been able to close some kind of gap? Have they engaged in some additional physical building of something in the heart, an action which required the help of the whole heart to pump more blood for its accomplishment? Such a project would definitely raise the pulse.

Then the thing is done. The heart goes back to its previous pace. It goes down as precipitately as it went up. Is this fantastic reasoning? Perhaps. But it will have to do until someone works out a better reason. Perhaps it was not the heart alone. Is it possible that my lungs were strengthening themselves, being able to perform more efficiently so as to give more oxygen to the heart with less physical action of taking breaths? Is it possible that on August 17 something physical happened with regard to my lungs, something that knitted together, something in which the heart had to take part by furnishing more blood for the building?

It is interesting to be aware that when a man-made machine has to be fixed, it must stop working, and outside forces do the job. But the heart performs the job of reconstruction itself and at the same time it pumps blood to the rest of the organs of the body.

One more observation. Beginning a few days ago, I noticed that the pulse during the second half minute of its taking goes down more than it used to. Before this, the pulse in the second period would be almost as high as that of the first. It indicates a newly acquired ability of the heart to snap back to normal after exertion. Another thing. I note that I breathe better while working at my desk.

I also wish to say that I can recommend the taking of vitamin E, based on a four-year detailed study of conservative medical researches regarding it. Like exercise, it oxygenates the tissues, and I have taken this vitamin in big doses for over ten years. The trouble with the average heart case no doubt is a stagnation within the body, a lack of circulating oxygen, due to a sedentary life.

During my daily walk, I perspire profusely. Perspiration is one means the body employs to get rid of toxins, or poisons. Is it possible that such poisons, remaining in the body because of a sedentary daily regimen, make the heart work harder to rid the body of them through other means and channels?

Is it also possible that these toxins by remaining in the body and distorting the blood chemistry on a permanent, continuing basis, further interfere with various internal processes, which throw additional strain onto the heart, thus forcing it to pump more rapidly in an attempt to reduce the condition?

There must be a reason why my pulse is going down, and I choose to think that a good sweat-out each day is part of it. By the sweat of thy brow shalt thou earn thy daily bread. Is this why farm workers are far less subject to heart disease than office-inhabiting men? Of course they exercise more, but

I think it is the combination of the two. Exercise breaks down old cells, causing new ones to form. It gives rise to an increase in the blood flow. Breathing is extended, and body functions stimulated. Muscles are kept in good repair, and their "tone" improved. There is a great improvement in the coordination of muscles and nerves. The circulation and elimination processes of the body are stimulated.

The late Dr. Raymond Pearl, of Johns Hopkins University, who studied the pulse records of thousands of individuals who died young, found that on the average their pulse rates were higher than normal. In the *Journal of the American Medical Association* of August 7, 1954, Drs. E. C. Hammond and D. Horn wrote the following: "A study conducted by the Society of Actuaries revealed that, among persons with a high pulse rate, the number of deaths from cancer was about 60 percent above the expected amount."

If you want to see an example of a heart shouting for help, examine my pulse readings for July 12, 13 and 14. A few weeks later I am able to do the same walk without the pulse once going over 100. It now looks as if it will be kept below 90 within a week or two. An hour a day of walking exercise must be a remarkable tonic to the body. I believe it is better than playing golf once or twice a week.

I was surprised, on August 1, 1954, to read in the Sunday *New York Times* magazine section that

Roger Bannister, who recently broke the one-mile running record, was able to do so by a method he used of reducing his pulse. "By making his heart a more muscular pump, he was able to reduce his pulse beat from its original 72 in repose to below 50," says this magazine.

By making his heart a more muscular pump! That must be what I am doing to mine.

Incidentally, my doctor, who examines my heart action and blood pressure once and sometimes twice a week, is quite satisfied with what he observes. Action is definitely improved, and my heart murmur is all but eliminated. Blood pressure which, when I began, was about 135/85, recently came down to 120/70, a figure which is well nigh perfect for any age and which I never had before that I can remember.

Not every heart case will be permitted to do what I have done. The physician must be the judge. Mine may be the ideal form of heart disease for this method of treatment. But there are more serious cases, and I would urge extreme caution. There are leaking hearts and oversized hearts. There are hearts damaged in various ways, and some that have had thrombosis, or blood clots. These people must depend on their physicians for guidance. I will say, however, that many individuals who have been suffering from a variety of heart ills and who have been immobilized, should have been set moving and working as soon as possible. I further believe that vitamin E can be a great insurance against a heart attack during these walks, but within the medical profession this is a subject of violent controversy. Why? I cannot understand.

What I have thus far done for my heart has two implications—one, I have built up the heart muscle: that is, improved the heart itself. Two, I have induced a condition in which the body can exercise with less effort, with less pumping on the part of the heart. Note also, in the extended tables, that the first reading which is the pulse at rest at home before starting on the daily walk, has gone down considerably. Eventually, this walking program may greatly reduce my "at rest" pulse. The other day I ran after a bus and was able to do it with the greatest of ease. There was no aftermath of pounding, nor the feeling that I might get a heart attack.

A few days ago I made a startling observation. My first heart symptoms had appeared in 1937, but it was in 1949 that they became really temperamental and troublesome. It was then that I had to increase my vitamin E dosage astronomically in order to relieve the chest pressure symptoms. I now know the reason why. A friend and I used to go on hikes, sometimes for eight or nine miles. It was in 1949 that he moved to Philadelphia and from then on I fell into a most sedentary routine—no long walks; and my heart rebelled.

I was told recently of a man who for 40 years was a track-walker for a railroad. For eight hours each day he walked the tracks to check for imperfections. A few years ago he retired and said, "Now I will rest." He then sat on his porch all day long. He was a healthy man, but within a year they laid him away to eternal rest. He had a heart attack. His heart could not stand the killing inactivity.

I look forward to these daily walking periods. It has become a time for thinking. One day when it rained and I could not walk I felt depressed about it all day, so that on a later day of inclement weather I went for my walk with an umbrella. It was a little difficult taking my pulse and holding the umbrella at the same time, but the actual readings were lower than for the previous day.

I also learned that foods of the average American diet raised my pulse from three to five points per minute. There were some that did not raise it at all, but when a food caused my pulse to run up eight or nine points it was one of the allergy-causing ones. In my own case I had a high pulse but no apparent allergies. Through years of study and analysis of my condition I was able to become so healthy that I no longer suffered from headaches or colds, and my blood pressure had gone down more or less to near normal. But it still was worthwhile to reduce my pulse.

I discovered that figs, honeydew melon, whole wheat, and fried foods of any kind were the basic troublemakers. It was absolutely fascinating running them down. For example, at first the indication showed that chicken raised my pulse unduly. But after I had accumulated sufficient records, showing in each case whether the chicken had been fried or broiled, I found that my pulse went up only when I ate fried chicken. I could eat broiled chicken without any trouble at all.

In the case of wheat, I made a rather thorough study. I found that whole wheat bread raised my pulse, but white bread did not. I could also eat wheat germ, which is present in whole wheat and not in white bread, without having the pulse go up. I therefore concluded that it was the bran that was difficult for my stomach to handle. This would indicate that, for me, the best kind of bread would be one with everything in it but the bran—a branless whole wheat bread. However, I found that I could eat raw wheat without raising the pulse.

French fried potatoes would send my pulse up, but not mashed or baked with the skins. It was the oil used in frying that I seemed to have difficulty in handling. I could eat cantaloupe but not honeydew, and regarding figs, I used to eat them by the pound. No wonder my pulse had been around 85 and sometimes 95. (Note: A few weeks ago I checked my pulse again on figs and found that now I could eat them without raising it. It may indicate a gradual strengthening of the body.)

I found that coffee did not raise my pulse even a point, and was surprised. I am not a regular drinker of alcoholic beverages but, just to test, I drank some scotch and soda and beer, and was amazed to find that such drinks also kept the pulse down.

Regarding coffee, I discovered that the way we made it, in glass, did not raise my pulse, but if boiled in an aluminum utensil it *did* raise it unduly. In this respect I would like to mention the fact that Dr Arthur E. Coca, in the book *The Pulse Test* (Arc Books Inc., New York, 1959), cites the cases of six patients whose pulses were raised by eating foods cooked in aluminum pots. Coca says, "Vaughan in his *Practice of Allergy,* p. 831, mentions 'the cure of cases of long-standing refractory colitis following change from aluminum cooking utensils to enamel or glass vessels.' "

Since there seems to be such a strong vegetarian movement and at times I have been tempted to try a vegetarian diet, I made sure to observe carefully the effect of meats on my pulse. In no case were they unfavorable. In other words, in my stomach, meat is digested very easily. It is a known medical fact, incidentally, that meat does not have to be chewed much. It is the carbohydrates that need lots of work in the mouth. Bear in mind, however, that these idiosyncrasies with regard to food vary with different persons. I may have an allergy to honeydew, for example, while you might eat it with impunity. So it is important that you check your own case thoroughly.

It is terrific in its implications when one considers what a reduction of the pulse actually means. In my own case the pulse was reduced by 15 points per minute. This means that every hour my pulse beat 60 × 15 or 900 times less. And in a full 24-hour day my heart had to expand and contract 900 × 24 less times or 21,600 less times a day. Merely by eliminating a few foods that I can easily get along without, my heart saves 43,200 movements in only one day. This is 21,600 expansions and 21,600 contractions. The heart actually moves between one and two inches each time in such expansion and contraction. Can you visualize this? Try and open and close your fist 21,600 times, moving it each time from one to two inches.

This means a saving of 15,768,000 movements a year for my little old heart. Is it any wonder that Dr. Raymond Pearl found that people who die young on the average have high pulses?

It certainly will pay everyone who reads this to check his or her pulse immediately, and if it is above 75 to try to discover what is raising it. In Coca's work he is able to bring patients' pulses down to as low as 65.

If you do decide to study your pulse, my suggestion is to note down the record of your pulse before and after each meal (one half hour and one hour after) for about one week so that you can have something to shoot at. After you have found the five or six offending foods that have been playing havoc with your pulse, you will note the effect of their elimination on the pulse recordings after full meals.

In my own case I had one extremely interesting

experience which is worth telling. Several times, my pulse went up after a meal more than it should have according to what I ate, and after thinking about it I discovered that at those meals I had forgotten to take my vitamins. I then proceeded to check on it by alternately taking my vitamins and leaving them out after meals, and it worked every time. It would indicate that the vitamins I was taking were aiding my digestion. This also shows that it was best for me to take my vitamins at my meals. I checked the effect of each vitamin separately. Some worked and others did not. But bone meal worked every time in keeping the pulse down.

In his book Coca describes symptoms which disappeared by lowering the pulse, in conditions of migraine, fatigue, nervousness, indigestion, dizziness, constipation, neuralgia, canker sores, chronic rhinitis, heartburn, urticaria, epileptic seizures, overweight, psychic depression, asthma and many others. It looks to me as if here we have a method that may revolutionize our entire conception of health and disease. Physicians should get a copy of Dr. Coca's work.

Shall we do away with labor-saving devices and the automobile? No! But let us keep moving as much as possible during our leisure hours. Let us form hiking groups for young and old.

Regarding vegetarians—many of them live long and I believe it is because they are generally health-conscious. A great many vegetarians are physical culturists, and know the value of exercise and walking. Witness the fantastic activities of

Bernard MacFadden when he was way above eighty.

I knew a vegetarian who lived to be 94. He would have lived to be 100 if he hadn't fallen out of a nut tree that he was pruning at the age of 92. He came to see me about five years ago and explained the value of his diet which was practically limited to fruits and nuts, but I believe it was his keeping on the move which was an important part of his formula for long living.

At the time of his visit to my farm he was 90 and spent most of his time prowling about the fields. He was more active than a barrel of monkeys, and if it had been pruning time, he would have "done" all our trees. I have to smile now when I recall him, but I was blind at the time, being lax on all forms of exercise. However, it is not too late.

Thus far I have stressed nutrition and physical movement. If we wish to live to be 90 or more I believe there should be added one more plank in the platform—something spiritual. Without it, not only would it be difficult to attain to a nonagenarian state, but you wouldn't want to. It would be boring. There must be a belief in the idealistic way a tolerance toward your fellow man, a lightness of spirit, a strong belief in God and a sense of humor. Given nutrition, movement and spirit, there would be far less of disease and far more of life.

My final advice to all—keep moving, but stay out of trees after you are 90.

CHAPTER XVII

The Story of Roseto, Pennsylvania

FROM SCIENTIFIC DISCOVERIES assembled from around the world, we have attempted to prove to you in this book that diseases of the heart and circulatory system are largely preventable. Many factors have been examined: fats in the diet and the difference between saturated and unsaturated fats; the role of carbohydrates in our diet, particularly the role of sugar; how vitamins and minerals function to maintain cardiovascular health; the harmful effect of certain drugs and other undesirable substances; and the benefits of exercise and weight control.

While diseases of the cardiovascular system are complicated, as we have seen, and there is much scientific controversy concerning which of the many factors is most crucial, we can nevertheless state with conviction: the road-signs to prevention are clear and simple! Modern living has brought about an epidemic of cardiovascular disease. It has removed essential elements from our food and added harmful elements. It has promoted a sedentary life that our systems were never meant to tolerate. But we have it in our power to overcome these obstacles. With care, our food can be "right," as nature intended it, and our life need not be confined to a desk and an easy chair.

The lesson that this book seeks to teach can best be illustrated in the story of Roseto, Pennsylvania. The little town of Roseto has received much publicity in recent years because of its remarkably low death rate due to heart disease. After journeying to Roseto to investigate, J. I. Rodale reported his findings in an article in *Prevention*, November, 1964. It is reproduced here as a fitting conclusion to this volume.

Perhaps you have been reading about a small town in eastern Pennsylvania called Roseto, which has a very low rate of heart disease deaths, (about half the national average), and where the people are very happy. This finding was discovered by Dr. Stewart Wolf, head of the University of Oklahoma's Department of Medicine, in 1962. When the news hit the newspapers, the theme seemed to be that these Rosetans were a very happy people, and therefore they lived long, and with less heart trouble.

Roseto is a community of 1,600 inhabitants, practically all Italians, who "know how to get fun out of life." There seems to be a happier atmosphere here, says Dr. Wolf. In Roseto people enjoy themselves. They are vigorous, comfortable and generally happier than anywhere else in the U. S. They really live!

In the usual American community, people engage in a kind of rat race, Dr. Wolf observes. "They don't have much emotional support from each other. Living is highly competitive—a constant keeping-up with the Joneses. Contrastingly, Roseto is a highly democratic town. Everyone has his place and appears to be pretty happy with what he has to do. Jobs people have are not much different from those in other communities, but social life is more pleasant."

As far as jobs are concerned the people work in the textile industry, many of the women working in shirt and blouse factories. Some of the men work in slate quarries. Others commute to Easton

	Population 1960	*Number of Deaths*	*Rate per/1000*
Roseto	1,630	11	6.7
Nazareth	6,209	71	11.5
Stroudsburg	6,070	97	16
Bangor	5,766	64	11.1
Pen Argyl	3,693	63	17.1
Wind Gap	1,930	27	13.9

(The rate for the entire U. S. is 9.5)

and Bethlehem to work in steel and other industries. Years ago, however, almost all the men worked in the slate quarries.

On page 224 are the death statistics for Roseto and a few neighboring towns for 1961.

The medical investigators are baffled since the Rosetans have more animal fat in their diets than most Americans, which would discredit the theory that saturated fat intake and heart disease are connected. The Philadelphia *Sunday Bulletin* (January 27, 1963) referred to the borough of Roseto as probably the most overweight community in the nation (a fact that Rosetans considered exaggerated).

The *Bulletin* went on to trace the town's history. Founded about 73 years ago by immigrants from Roseto, Italy, it quickly became close-knit, because the newcomers were rejected by the older settlers of the area. Many of the newcomers were related. Forced together, they wove a web of mutual concern and friendship. Dr. Wolf said, "We found a happier atmosphere in Roseto than in most communities because people here like each other."

For several years, on and off, Dr. Wolf and his staff examined most of the adult population of the town, and their report of it appears in the June 8, 1964, issue of the *Journal of the American Medical Association.*

The article speaks of the way the Rosetans seem to enjoy life, being gay, and boisterous, but unpretentious. They are simple, warm and very hospitable people. They were found to be mutually trusting, and without any criminal tendencies, there being very little crime in Roseto.

The article states that obesity and a generous consumption of calories, fat and wine were actually associated with a strikingly low death rate from myocardial infarction, a form of heart attack.

To give an example of the comparison of this form of heart attack in Roseto with four other nearby towns, a table is given of the death rate from this condition per 100,000 of population, averaging the seven years from 1955-1961, as follows:

Roseto	157
Nazareth	603
Bangor	613
Stroudsburg	671
East Stroudsburg	405

According to the article, the cholesterol in the Rosetans is about the same as in other Americans. The doctors state, therefore, that this is not a factor in producing the low Rosetan death rate.

As far as dietary habits are concerned, "a favorite dish, *prosciuto*, a pressed ham delicacy, has a rim of fat more than an inch thick and the Rosetans eat it whole without discarding the fat . . . cooking is done by most families with lard rather than olive oil . . . and most dipped their bread in the gravy to consume the whole dish."

The article winds up by saying that the reason for the low death rate from myocardial infarction in Roseto is not very clear, and is still to be determined.

When the first account of the situation in Roseto appeared in the newspapers I read about it with avid interest, but I questioned the idea that they are living long because they are a very happy people. I recalled the case of the Hunzas of Northern India (see my book *The Healthy Hunzas*, 1948). They too are a very happy people, with practically no crime. But it has been shown that they are happy because they are healthy, and not healthy because they are happy. I decided it would be necessary for me to go to Roseto and see what I could observe.

It being only about 40 miles from Allentown, my wife and I went there in the summer of 1963, and we have been there several times since. The first thing that hit me was the fact that there are so many steep, hilly streets in this town. This has not been mentioned anywhere in the dozens of news items I have seen about Roseto, or in the *Journal of the American Medical Association* article mentioned. But walking up and down hills from childhood can be a terrific factor in the health picture. And these older Italians brought the habit of walking from the old country.

Walking uphill increases the specific gravity of the tissues of the body, which enables the whole body, including the heart, to operate more efficiently. A high specific gravity means that the tissues are more compact. There is more weight to each cubic inch of body tissue.

Walking and exercising generally reduces the blood pressure and the pulse. I would suggest that, in their continuing work, Dr. Wolf and his staff take specific gravity and blood pressure readings in the five cities. It may show a decided difference between Roseto and the other towns. I would suggest also a comparison of pulse readings in the five towns. Dr. Raymond Pearl of Johns Hopkins proved that on the average, the higher the pulse the shorter the life.

Talking about hill walking, there is a sanitorium in Bad Nauheim, Germany, which specializes in heart cases. It makes use of three long hills, one with a 5 percent grade, the second with a 10 percent grade, and the third with a grade of 15 percent. The patient is gradually conditioned until he can walk the 15 percent grade with ease, and it has been found to strengthen the heart.

I walk an hour a day in a hilly section. When I spent one winter at Palm Beach, which is very flat, and where we lived in a one-story house, with no stair-climbing, my blood pressure went up 30 points. A few weeks after I returned, my blood pressure went back to normal.

If these Rosetans did not walk these hills, they would be even more obese, their blood pressure and pulse would be higher, specific gravity lower, and their cholesterol still higher, for it is known that cholesterol is lowered by exercise. A high degree of obesity, on their high fat diet, with no exercise. would reduce their life-span.

In one of the newspaper accounts about Roseto (Allentown, Pa. *Call,* October 6, 1963), is shown a picture of the contented face of Joseph Trilli, aged 94. The caption reads, "Enjoying good health, the nonagenarian can be seen taking his daily walk." The older Rosetans like to walk. I was talking to a grocer whose place is on top of a hill. He said that most of his customers walked up the hill two or three times a day to get their groceries. He said, "The older people walk, but the younger people, if they have to go five blocks, ride." The older citizens worked harder. Roseto was dug out of a chestnut forest by hand. They had no bulldozers.

Point number two is something that I had a hunch about, as soon as I heard about these healthy Italians. Most of them raised their own vegetables, and many of them kept chickens so they not only consumed fresh food, but most important of all, I found that very few people in Roseto used chemical fertilizers or poisonous insecticides. They were following the organic method of gardening without knowing it by name. It was a tradition with their people in the old country which they brought with them. This is a tradition-loving people as I could see from the names of the streets in the town—Garibaldi, Columbus, Dante, etc. In the old country, anyone who had even a pocket handkerchief-sized piece of land who didn't grow vegetables was akin to a renegade, and it is the same in the American Roseto. But neither place depended on chemicals.

I needn't go into the subject too deeply, but food raised organically has more vitamins and minerals than food grown with chemical fertilizers, although the *Journal of the American Medical Association* has violently attacked this idea, writing articles so riddled with inaccuracies and omissions that it isn't even funny. We have published a booklet giving evidence only by physicians that organically raised food is more healthful than that raised by the usual chemical method.

In Roseto, my wife and I went from garden to garden—every house had one, and we saw only one that used a mild form of chemicals, but a neighbor told us that it was the case of an Italian woman married to an outsider. These people use manure as their fertilizer medium. Today the number of gardens has been reduced, unfortunately for Rosetans.

So, we have here a people who move about in hilly streets, and who raise a good part of their food in their own backyards in a wholesome manner. Now, how about their diet generally?

I can refer to the tradition of breast-nursing which was brought from the old country. The medical statistics prove that people who have been breast-nursed for a considerable period are the healthier for it. The doctors should check the trend today among the young folks in Roseto. Are they keeping up this tradition? What is the incidence of breast-nursing in Roseto as compared to the four towns?

While on the subject of breast-nursing let's consider milk, and the part it plays in the Rosetan diet. It will be found that they drink far less milk than the people in the other four towns. The Italians drink wine and their is practically a complete absence of milk drinking, in the older people. On a trip to Rome and Palermo recently, I noted that milk is used so little compared to the U. S., that it is sold in tobacco shops.

I spoke to older people in Roseto. Several of them told me they never drank milk at all. The old generation even dipped bread in wine and fed it to babies. Today, I am told, this is no longer done. Babies get more store milk and eat boxed cereals.

The older people were more frugal. They wouldn't eat ice cream except on rare occasions. In other words their total consumption of dairy products is far less than that of the neighboring towns. Now if I had the space I could give you 30 or 40 medical references to show that milk is *not* a healthful food for adults. It not only produces allergies in an enormous number of people, but recently it was found that children get nutritional anemia by overconsumption of milk, and an article in *Nutrition Reviews* (April, 1963) stated that some athletic coaches found that milk-drinking impairs prolonged athletic performance. I can give you dozens of references indicting milk-drinking as the cause of various disease conditions.

But the most amazing thing of all is that excessive milk-drinking in children increases their stature. That is why our youth today are growing into giants, a condition which is not desirable. Very tall people do not live as long as shorter-statured ones.

In Dr. Wolf's article in the *Journal of the American Medical Association* charts are given showing that the Rosetans are shorter in height. The Italians generally are very short people. So are the French. This is due to the fact that they drink very little milk, preferring wine. On my visits to Roseto I noticed how short the people were—much shorter than the people in the other four towns. But I did notice some very tall young Rosetan adults, who no doubt had been reading or were told that milk is a healthful food. They no doubt are also eating a lot of ice cream.

I recommend to Dr. Wolf that he study this milk factor, and that his staff make a thorough study of the medical literature on the subject to get at the truth about milk.

The Rosetans, old and young, do eat cheese, but as most Italians do, prefer the low-fat cheeses.

Now let's take the bread favored by the Rosetans. It is the typical Italian white bread made locally with far fewer chemical additives in it. For example, it does not contain any anti-staling chemicals, will stay soft much longer. The fact of the matter is that in the diet of the average Rosetan there is much less of chemical additives. They don't patronize the T. V. dinner, consume very little of canned foods, and won't go for frozen beef. They want local butchers to dress it. Bologna is made in Roseto without using any sodium nitrate as a preservative. They consume more raw foods and fresh fruit. It is a custom from the old country. The medical people should attempt to compare the amount of chemical additives consumed in an average daily diet in the five towns.

Another aspect about their diet is covered in a letter to me from C. B. Axford of New York City. He says: "Can it be possible that the researcher—Dr. Stewart Wolf of the University of Oklahoma—missed the obvious reason? Out of my acquaintance with some Roseto folk, and their fare, I suggest you look into the relatively large amount of garlic which Rosetans consume. This is one great dietetic difference between Roseto and the neighboring towns with which Dr. Wolf attempted to compare it.

"How's about your making a little supplementary study and giving the facts to Dr Wolf? Garlic's medicinal values are well known folk medicine among the Roseto oldsters."

American doctors don't think much of garlic but European researchers show that it can reduce high blood pressure, and is a natural antibiotic. Many opera stars eat garlic, claiming it prevents them from getting sore throats.

Then the wine of the Rosetans! The grapes for it are home grown. I saw garden after garden with their rows of grapevines, growing organically, without chemical fertilizers or poison sprays. The Rosetans make the wine themselves, using no chemical additives. The wine you buy has been treated with various chemical compounds for various purposes.

Again I say, the big thing with these Rosetans is that they get very little of the chemical additives which the average American has to ingest in his food every day.

Now, since they depend mainly on wine, the oldsters rarely drink soda pop or colas which have such a high sugar content. In the surrounding areas, however, large amounts of sugarized soda pop are consumed, and this is a point worth studying in connection with the Rosetan longevity and immunity to heart attacks.

I would like to say a few words about these youngsters in Roseto. They are not following the Italian ways with the intensity of their parents. They are eating more sweets, candies and refined foods. They don't go in as much for breast-nursing in their children. They drink milk and eat ice cream. Many of these young people own cars and get less exercise. They are taller and not as healthy as the older people. I was told they catch colds easily. I wonder if the average newly married youngsters arrange to do their own vegetable gardening.

Therefore, when the day of reckoning comes 30 or 40 years from now, will they live as long as the oldsters? Will Roseto be a medical experiment to show the effect on human health of the old and the new ways?

The Philadelphia *Sunday Bulletin,* January 27, 1963, had an article on Roseto with a big headline above it: "The Secret of Long Life in Roseto: Take it Easy, Eat, Get Fat, be Happy." After having read my article you can see how wrong this advice is. If you want to live long, don't rush to Roseto. You can have a Roseto in your own backyard, where you can have an organic garden. And if you have a choice, pick a hilly area in which to live. Walk an hour a day and do calisthenics. Don't live in a ranch-type one-story house. Don't drink milk or eat dairy foods, cut out sugared soft drinks and refined foods, candies, pies, cakes, etc., and everything packaged or canned that contains chemical additives. Then you can look forward to living as long as do the Rosetans.

Index

D

E

F

H

L

M

N

INDEX

O

P

R

S

T

V